HOW WE DIE NOW

KARLA A. ERICKSON

How We Die Now

*Intimacy and the Work
of Dying*

TEMPLE UNIVERSITY PRESS · PHILADELPHIA

TEMPLE UNIVERSITY PRESS
Philadelphia, Pennsylvania 19122
www.temple.edu/tempress

Library of Congress Cataloging-in-Publication Data

Erickson, Karla A., 1973–
 How we die now : intimacy and the work of dying / Karla A. Erickson.
    p. ; cm.
 Includes bibliographical references and index.
 ISBN 978-1-4399-0823-5 (cloth : alk. paper) — ISBN 978-1-4399-0824-2 (pbk. :
alk. paper) — ISBN 978-1-4399-0825-9 (e-book)
 I. Title.
 [DNLM: 1. Aged—psychology—United States.   2. Attitude to Death—United
States.   3. Death—United States.   4. Health Services for the Aged—United
States.   5. Intergenerational Relations—United States.   6. Residential Facilities—
United States. WT 116]
 R726.8
 362.17'5—dc23

                                                                      2013013287

∞ The paper used in this publication meets the requirements of the American
National Standard for Information Sciences—Permanence of Paper for Printed
Library Materials, ANSI Z39.48-1992

Printed in the United States of America

2 4 6 8 9 7 5 3 1

For my dad,

Darrell Rodney Erickson—

I miss you.

Contents

Acknowledgments

This book has been seven years in the making, and along the way I have incurred many debts. First, I thank all the people who make up Winthrop House for embracing this project, as they embrace so many other aspects of living and aging. From the beginning, residents, workers, and administrators at Winthrop House welcomed me and encouraged this investigation, and that has made all the difference.

Next, I thank Grinnell College for the generous award of two one-year research leaves—one when I was a junior faculty member and one after I received tenure—to pursue all the promising leads and follow the many paths generated by this study. Time to think and write is a form of wealth in academe, and I have been generously granted such time. Thanks also go to Richard Fyffe, librarian of Grinnell College, who made certain that both resources and silence were readily available to me by providing an office in the library during my two years of research. De Dudley supported the project with administrative help at every stage. I am also grateful to the students who accompanied me at various times during the study. Jenny Weber and Eszter Csicsai helped me shape the project from the start. Alyssa Penner, Margie Scribner, Kate Howard, John Burrows, Virginia Anderson, Macaela Holmes, and Nichole Baker informed aspects of the project by developing relationships at Winthrop House. Ragnar Thorisson and Liting Cong conducted international comparative research that helped me situate the specific dynamics of American aging and dying processes. Nichole Baker, Malory Dreasler, Gina Physic, and especially Maia Pillot did the thankless work of transcribing the interviews for this project, and Sunanda Vaidheesh worked as a research assistant hunting down numerous sources for me.

I thank my sister, Kate Erickson, and my mom, Cathie Corcoran, who assisted me with this project, as they do with all my life's projects, by offering advice on multiple versions of the manuscript. I also benefited enormously from the support and constructive criticism provided by friends and colleagues in two writing groups. David Cook-Martin, Dan Reynolds, and Astrid Henry, as members of the book club, helped usher this project from its infancy. And Shanna Benjamin, Angela Onwuachi-Willig, Lakesia Johnson, and Michelle Nasser, as members of the women's writing group, kept my feet to the fire to ensure that I saw the project through. I am so lucky to have such brilliant, generous critics. Finally, I thank my former adviser and lifelong friend, Jennifer Pierce, who taught me how to conduct ethnography and how to write books—without her, I would not have pursued this career, which challenges and sustains me.

At Temple University Press, I thank Mick Gusinde-Duffy, who recognized potential in this project early in its development and helped shape its final form. Editors who talk on the level of ideas and audience and who take the time to truly understand a project are rare; I am grateful to have found such an editor in

Mick. When Mick departed for a new job, Micah Kleit stepped in to finish the project, and Gary Kramer and his skilled associates marketed the book. Nanette Bendyna smoothed the text and details with her skilled copyediting, and Tom Annese created the index. Closer to home, Dan Weeks, Grinnell College editor, passionately conveyed the message of the book to local audiences.

At home, I thank my husband, Matthew Karjalahti, who keeps me grounded, laughing, and curious. And I give a loving welcome to our new son, Erikson Karjalahti, whose birth enlivened my study of old age and death and whose life is a source of joy for his dad and me. Matthew and Erikson both help me make sense of our little place on the planet.

HOW WE DIE NOW

I

⸎

How We Die Now

Americans Aging and Dying
in the Twenty-First Century

I n the spring of 2002, I met Sarah, a hospice nurse caring for
my grandmother, Phyllis Walsh, during one of the last days
of her life. Grandma Phyllis was in her seventies when cancer
infested her body. After several months of caring for her at home,
Grandpa, my mom, my sister, and I were relieved when Grandma
Phyllis qualified for hospice care. In the quiet and peaceful hospice
wing of the hospital near her home in the Twin Cities, we were
able to enjoy Grandma's final days rather than scramble to try to
care for her at home. At home, we had scrambled to adapt to her
changing needs, struggled to lift and clean her pained body, and
failed too often to protect her pride and privacy. We loved her, but
we were out of our element and sometimes over our heads trying
to care for her. In hospice, we could leave the skilled part of her
care to the nurses and focus on making the most of our remaining
time together. I even had the privilege of witnessing Grandpa and
Grandma saying good-bye to each other. When Phyllis started to
move into the final stages of death, the members of our extended

family were able to gather and talk to her and among ourselves, knowing that her physical needs were being addressed by the remarkable nurses who worked in the hospice wing.

During those final days, we practically lived on the hospice wing, and it was then that I witnessed Sarah doing her amazing work. During one eight-hour shift, I observed Sarah touch and turn bodies, raise beds, massage limbs, chart physical changes, measure pain, treat symptoms, and dress wounds. In addition to offering the physical strength, stamina, and medical knowledge that she clearly possessed, Sarah took care of the emotional and spiritual needs of her patients and their families. She acted as a mediator for members of a family who had not spoken to one another for over a decade, discussed with a granddaughter of one of her patients whether or not angels existed, and encouraged an elderly man to let his wife "go" now. As someone who studies work and identity, I was mesmerized by how demanding, multifaceted, and important Sarah's labor was. The intellectual, physical, spiritual, and emotional work that Sarah did in those eight hours was, to my mind, beyond the realm of remuneration. How would you prepare a worker to be thrown suddenly into a pivotal moment in the history of a family? How would you train someone to be responsible for teaching about death at the moment of dying? These are some of the questions that inspired this study.

As a hospice nurse, Sarah received special training in palliative care and helping others die. Unlike Sarah, most individuals who grapple with the changes of old age are *not* trained to do so, including home health workers, nurse's aides in nursing homes, family care providers, and even many doctors, who often learn how to help others navigate the end of life through trial and error. Trained or not, these workers help others die, and in the process they learn about their patients and themselves, and about living and dying.

As an ethnographer of labor, I investigate why workers are attracted to their work, what they learn from their work, and what sustains and challenges them. I wrote this book because I wanted to know what the "Sarahs" of the world knew: I wanted to know more about aging and dying and to be comfortable in that knowledge. I wanted mortality to be less hidden, more familiar. I interviewed and observed many "Sarahs"—true end-of-life experts—for this book. I recount their stories here to inform and inspire the rest of us, who find ourselves navigating a changing landscape of old age and death for which we have no training and little preparation to encounter.

Demography Is Destiny

In 2011, the United States lurched over the starting line of a seismic demographic shift that scholars refer to as global aging (Angel and Angel 1997; Kiernan 2006). Many of the readers of this book will witness the peak of this change during their lifetimes. Consider this snapshot of how dramatically the balance between youth and old age will change. In the year 2000, just over a decade ago, the number of centenarians—people over the age of one hundred—in the whole world was 180,000. In one decade, that number has more than doubled, having grown to 450,000. By 2050, that number is expected to increase even more rapidly to an estimated 3.2 million humans over one hundred years of age (Fishman 2010: 8). This substantial rise in the number of centenarians is just one of the demographic puzzle pieces that will significantly change cultures around the world in the coming decades. Some demographers tell us that by 2050 older people will outnumber children for the first time in human history (United Nations 2008). This transition began in the United States in 2011, when the first of the baby boomers[1] turned sixty-five years of age, moving the United States ever closer to a society in which old age and death are more common than birth and childhood.

The average number of children born has dropped dramatically as well over the last forty years. For example, in the United States, the average birthrate dropped from 3.1 children in 1975 to 1.9 in 2005, producing a sharp rise in the proportion of Americans over age sixty-five relative to younger Americans (Korczyk 2004). Urbanization, availability of reliable birth control, and the employment of many more women have combined to reduce the number of children born while increasing the total number of people in the workforce. For several decades the proliferation of women in the workplace masked the declining number of available workers; now, as both women and men "age out" of the workforce, the shifting balance between active workers and retirees becomes clear. Take, for example, the case of Spain, which currently has one of the oldest populations in the world. The aging of the population in Spain is also produced by a combination of longer lives and lower fertility rates; however, the pace of elongated lives and declining birthrates is faster and further along than in other European nations. Currently, life expectancy in Spain is 83.8 years for women, the highest in Europe, and 77.2 years for men ("Aging Population in Spain" 2007). Meanwhile, the average birthrate dropped dramatically from 3.0 children in 1975 to just 1.2 children today, one of the lowest birthrates in the world. Demographers predict that these two forces, taken together, will produce a 24 percent decline in the Spanish population by 2050. By that same year, Spain will have the highest percentage of elder people in the world. People sixty-five and older will constitute 37 percent of the population by

---

1. Baby boomers are individuals who were born between 1946 and 1965 (Howe and Strauss 1991).

that date, an increase of 117 percent over the current percentage (Bosch 2000).

Nations vary in how they approach the graying of the population. Currently, the vast majority—85 percent—of retired people in Spain reside with family, but institutional care is becoming a more popular alternative (Botsford 2002). This low rate of institutional care is in contrast to that of Norway, for example, "where home care has been available for over 25 years. There, surveys show, old people prefer *not* to have family members provide personal care" (Neysmith and Aronson 1996: 13; italics added). In the United States, the oldest old are the most likely to live in institutionalized care settings such as nursing homes. While not every nation deals with the changing balance of youth and old age in the same way, many will face decisions in the coming decades about how to provide care and support to an elderly cohort that is quickly outnumbering its younger counterparts.

Taken together, the demographic changes in average birthrate and average life expectancy alter what demographers call the dependency ratio. The dependency ratio is a calculation of the proportion of the working population who can support those who are not in the labor force.

> Commonly, the dependency ratio relates to the number of people who are unproductive because of age (under 15 and over 65 years of age), because of infirmity, or because they are involved in an organized activity such as child rearing, to those who are productive, usually employers or employees between the ages of 15 and 65. (Baltes 1996: 13)

The dependency ratio is one way of capturing the shifting balance between youth and old age in a culture. This ratio is a critical measure for social planning because it "indicates the locations along the age spectrum at which there are more dependents than working producers" (Baltes 1996: 13). The dependency ratio can also help calculate the needed level of contributions for programs like social security, and it can provide a glimpse into the caregiving demands faced on average by a particular generation. For example, in the United States, "some analysts estimate that this situation will worsen: baby boomers probably will put in, on average, 18 years assisting elders as compared to 17 raising their children" (Olson 2003: 56). What will it mean to live in a world in which seventy years of age is more common than ten years of age? What will we need to change about our social infrastructure to accommodate those changes? And, given our longer lives and slower deaths, who should care for us and how? These are just some of the questions that arise as a result of the dramatic demographic changes under way.

The Longevity Dividend

In the twenty-first century, many of us are living longer, dying slower, and, more importantly, dying *differently* than our ancestors. The territories of old age and dying have changed greatly in only a few generations. Many humans born today will live as many as thirty years longer than their ancestors. Around the world, the average life expectancy in 1900 was thirty years of age. By 2000, that average had risen to sixty-four (Fishman 2010: 13). Worldwide, better nutrition and health care combined with technological advances in medical care have extended longevity. As Ted Fishman explains, if you add up all the extra years of life, "today's 6.7 billion people will enjoy more than 250 billion extra years of life" than if we had been born just a century ago (2010: 13). Through medicinal advancements, new technologies, and lifestyle alterations, Americans born today have a life expectancy thirty years longer than that of previous generations (United Nations 2008). In the United States, average life expectancy was forty-seven at the turn of the last century, rising to seventy-seven in 2000 (U.S. Bureau of the Census 2010). Some scholars describe this extra time as the "longevity dividend" and the "true wealth of nations" (United Nations 2008).

The longevity dividend is the combined result of two changes: longer lives and slower deaths. At both societal and individual levels, many adjustments will have to be made to accommodate and seize the potential offered by the longevity dividend. If societies prepare and lay claim to the opportunity, the longevity dividend offers the potential for longer, richer, fuller lives. However, the longevity dividend could also be squandered if societies do not anticipate and prepare for the eminent demographic changes by altering social structures and becoming informed about the needs and possibilities that arise from living and working in an aged society.

The first force producing greater longevity is that many fatal diseases have been modified or eliminated by modern medicine. Many diseases that once caused immediate death can now be managed for many additional years of life or even cured altogether. Many more humans have access to safe, abundant, and reliable food, safe sewage removal, and potable drinking water. Medical science has better informed our understanding of how disease is transmitted, and changes in personal hygiene and public health have responded to this new knowledge. Preventive medicine has improved, as has the ability to extend life once a disease has been diagnosed. Taken together, all these changes have added up to longer lives.

The second force shaping longevity is that dying processes in the contemporary era are now incremental as compared to the more sudden deaths most humans experienced in the past

(Kiernan 2006: 7). For example, in the United States, strokes and accidents have been replaced as the top killers. Americans now die from slower, longer diseases, including cancer, heart disease, and Alzheimer's disease (Kiernan 2006: xv). This is not to say that sudden deaths no longer occur from childbirth, car accidents, or heart attacks, but rather it is more common for people to die after a slow decline due to multiple chronic diseases. These shifts have resulted in a dramatic social change: contemporary humans can now see their own death coming. "The change, for a growing number of people every day, is this: dying today is gradual. For the first time in human history, we can anticipate our mortality. We can watch its slow approach. We can look it in the eye" (Kiernan 2006: 12). The prolonged process of dying that now characterizes many end-of-life experiences opens up new opportunities that are easily overlooked because of a lack of preparation.

Our social rituals and the social organization of old age and death have not kept pace with our longer lives and slower deaths. As Dr. Atul Gawande explains, longer lives introduce more time, but that time is often accompanied by uncertainty and even confusion about what differentiates life from death.

> For all but our most recent history, dying was typically a brief process. Whether the cause was childhood infection, difficult childbirth, heart attack, or pneumonia, the interval between recognizing that you had a life-threatening ailment and death was often just a matter of days or weeks. These days, for most people, death comes only after long medical struggle with an incurable condition—advanced cancer, progressive organ failure or the multiple debilities of very old age. In all such cases, death is certain, but the timing isn't. So everyone struggles with this uncertainty—with how, and when, to accept that the battle is

lost. Technology sustains our organs until we are well past the point of awareness and coherence. (Gawande 2010: 38)

Unlike sudden and rapid deaths, which created a short period of dying (sometimes minutes, sometimes weeks or months), the new conditions of dying often result in years of ups and downs, of good days and bad, and of prolonged dying processes for which we do not yet have rituals, best practices, or even the language to describe. Dr. Gawande explains, "In the past few decades, medical science has rendered obsolete centuries of experience, tradition, and language about our mortality, and created a new difficulty for mankind: how to die" (2010: 40). As such, although prolonged dying offers many possible benefits, as a historically new phenomenon, it also entails confusion and concern.

Along with the remarkable inheritance of longer lives come the challenges that accompany rapid social change, including worse health, longer illnesses, slower deaths, longer aging, and increased dementia. As Daniel Callahan explains, "Death now principally comes from the chronic and degenerative diseases of aging." The dying process is also shaped now by what Callahan calls "technological brinkmanship" (1993: 40–47). Brinkmanship is defined as the "art or practice of pushing a dangerous situation or confrontation to the limit of safety especially to force a desired outcome" (Merriam Webster Dictionary Online 2010). Technological brinkmanship is fed by forces in the medical system, including how doctors are trained, the litigiousness of medicine, and the separation of science and ethics. As Janet Shim, Ann Russ, and Sharon Kaufman explain, doctors are trained to assess if a patient meets the criteria for a procedure. If the patient does, then the procedure is encouraged. Physicians are not keen to advise against a procedure because doing so would reveal their estimates about how long a patient has to live, and "who wants to be part of that [possible] miscalculation?" (2006). Treating illness with procedures takes on an imperative without regard to quality of life. That imperative replaces choice and deliberation. More invasive procedures make additional procedures conceivable, and so the path of endless intervention begins.

Technological brinkmanship prolongs life, but the attendant danger is the lack of quality that might accompany such prolongations. On the positive side, prolonged dying offers the opportunity to wrap up one's life deliberately, to fulfill final wishes, to say good-bye to loved ones, even to plan one's own funeral. On the negative side, prolonged dying presents the dying person and his or her family members with historically new options for which there is no clear ethical or social road map. Is prolonging life good regardless of quality? How do we plan younger lives around the ups and downs of older lives? Dying individuals and their family members have to make difficult decisions that can induce uncertainty, confusion, hurt feelings, and shame.

Despite this future toward which we are rushing, many of us approach it seriously underprepared to face death personally or professionally. This book uses the experiences of workers, residents, family members of patients, and administrators at a continuing care retirement community (CCRC) that I call Winthrop House. I use the experience and knowledge of these people to help explore the new conditions of old age and the when and why of how we die now. What could be learned from end-of-life workers about accompanying others toward death? Might we find ourselves better prepared for death, or even better able to live, if we confront what they know? These were the questions with which I began this study. Despite the potential of the longevity dividend, currently our social, economic, and medical systems are mismatched with the conditions of our longer lives and slower deaths. The remainder of the book explains the fears and anxieties that currently lock us into mismatched approaches and responds to these fears with the knowledge and insights of end-of-life workers. I believe that we can learn from the expertise of individuals whose jobs require them to be flexible, facile, and creative in the face of new social facts.

Longevity and Inequality

The longevity dividend is not equally distributed. The final chapter of life is shaped by the gender, race, and class-based systems of privilege and oppression that structure the rest of life. First, the longevity dividend is a privilege of the young and the accident of being born in an advanced industrialized country. The youngest generation has the longest life expectancy in almost all nations (with the exception of war-torn nations); however, the life expectancy varies widely *across* nations. As Ted Fishman makes clear, being born into an advanced industrialized nation is the biggest contributor to longevity.

> If you look across history, at every culture that ever existed, reviewing all the scientific literature and self-help books, you find only one crack-sure mode of maximum life extension: it is best to be born sometime after the turn of the twentieth century, preferably, though not necessarily, in an affluent, developed country. Nothing else even comes close. (2010: 70)

Within nations, life expectancy also varies by race, class, and gender. Each of these factors influences the kind of choices available to elders, the quality of care received, and the likelihood of needing assistance in one's later years. So while the longevity dividend is a shared social phenomenon, individual experiences are influenced by one's social location.

In nineteenth- and twentieth-century American culture, care of the aged and the dying was defined as women's work that women should and usually did provide for free to their blood relatives and their husbands' relatives. In the twenty-first century, caring for dependents continues to be women's work, both paid and unpaid. Care for the aged and dying is not recognized as difficult physical and psychological work that is financially straining, and even spiritually draining. When elder care moves into the public sphere, it remains encoded as women's work, and it is primarily women—particularly women of color—who are poorly paid to care for dependent elders, be it in home health care, nursing homes, or CCRCs (Glenn 2010). In fact, women make up a whopping 77 percent of the adult children providing care to elderly parents, and 60 percent of women will provide private elder care at some point in their lives (Margolies 2004; Olson 2003).

In the United States, not only are women the caregivers; they are also the most likely to be the *recipients* of institutional care: women make up 65 percent of all residents in nursing homes (U.S. Bureau of the Census 2009). Because women, regardless of race or class, live longer than men on average and marry people older than themselves on average, they are more likely than men to be widowed. Even if they are still alive, husbands are also less likely than women to care for their spouses at home. As a result of all these tendencies, women are the primary recipients of institutionalized care. Elder women are also more likely to live alone at the end of their lives: among white women aged sixty-five to seventy-five, 33 percent live alone as compared with only 12 percent of white men (Olson 2003: 103). This disparity continues and increases as white men and women age. By the age of eighty-five, a startling 59 percent of white women and 28 percent of white men live alone. White men are more likely to have unpaid care in their homes from wives, daughters, or other female relatives, while white women are more likely to find themselves alone and potentially in need of institutional care. Black women are even more likely to be single than white women of the same age, and since older black people are three times as likely to be impoverished and have approximately half the wealth of white people of the same age, black elders are less likely to have a range of choices for addressing their needs in the later years of life (Olson 2003: 133).

In short, white people are more likely to live longer and to have real choices about the conditions of their care in their final years and days. The privileges of being white and the relative disadvantage of being black, Latin American, American Indian, or Asian American accumulate over time. Laura Katz Olson explains how these different experiences take shape over the life course and are incorporated in health outcomes and care regimens. "Minority and other deprived older populations, who have suffered a lifetime of poverty, poor nutrition, and limited access to medical care, tend to have greater mortality, morbidity, disabling conditions, and inferior health status overall than the more advantaged groups" (2003: 9). Rather than being influenced by just the aging process per se, longevity, frailty, and dependency are all shaped by social, economic, cultural, and political contexts.

In the United States, the longevity dividend is largely shaped by structural racism. For example, even our life horizon—average life expectancy—is deeply divided by race. In the United States, current life expectancies for a white woman and a white man are 80.8 and 75.9 years, respectively, while the average life expectancy for a black woman is 77.4 years and for a black man 70.9, a full decade less than for a white woman (Centers for Disease Control and Prevention 2011). Racial minority elders are more invisible, more likely to be poor, and more likely to live with members of their extended family in the final years of life. Amazingly, even pain management varies by racial category. "Physical pain among the dying remains uncontrolled, often unaddressed, and certain groups of people are at much greater risk than others. In America, you have a greater chance of dying in pain if you don't speak English, and if you are black, Hispanic, poor, elderly, or a woman" (Byock 1997: 242).

Finally, while minority elders are more likely to *need* assistance at the end of their lives, they are less likely to make use of institutional care. Many minority elders express distrust in institutionalized elder care, and in many minority communities, the expectation that younger generations will care for the old is very strong, making family care the obvious choice. Given the long history of systematic institutional neglect and abuse of black Americans—such as the Tuskegee experiments in which black men were intentionally given syphilis, the widespread forced sterilization of black women by doctors, and the failure to study and address ailments that disproportionately affect black communities—black elders have reason to proceed with caution when seeking long-term care (Allott and Robb 1998). Many black families are reluctant to turn over the care of their loved ones to institutional care. Social science research also suggests that minority filial networks are stronger than white ones, in part as a means of surviving and thriving in a racist culture divided by social class. As Olson explains, "For Blacks, Latinos, and Asians, whose values emphasize collectivism, interdependence, and mutual assistance the dependency of frail older people on their family is both expected and accepted as a predictable phase of the life cycle" (2003: 127–128). In short, minority Americans' "preference" for family care likely reflects family values and also potentially exposes disparate access to for-pay services. As the elder boom develops, formal and informal decisions about how to make use of the longevity dividend will determine if inequality continues to characterize the final chapter of our lives.

Dilemmas of the Threshold

I call the challenges and opportunities afforded by these new social conditions of old age dilemmas of the threshold. I use the notion of a threshold to describe the ambiguity of the space between living and dying that has become a more common experience. This threshold is the liminal space between living and dying. Unlike sudden deaths, prolonged dying produces a period of time—sometimes days, sometimes years—when one is living with chronic diseases that are deadly but that have not yet resulted in death. Because this kind of dying is protracted, it is neither a time of dying nor a time of living as in other stages of life because it is haunted by the eminence of death. Both the dying persons and those around them struggle to know how to behave during this time and have no real social map to follow. This is not a time to gather and grieve at a bedside because it is not active dying; rather, it is the accumulation of wear and tear on old bodies combined with chronic diseases that makes death foreseeable but not predictable. So I use the concept of a threshold to describe this time: like standing on the threshold of a door frame between two rooms—one room is living without the specter of dying, the other room is death itself. Eventually, one will have to walk forward into death, but the time for that next step is unknown.

The sudden deaths that were prevalent in previous eras provided little warning, but they did have the advantage of clarity. When death was sudden, it was accompanied by harsh and incontrovertible recognition that the end of life was near. Sudden deaths were like a light switch: a person switched from actively living to actively dying. Sudden deaths left little time for goodbyes, recognition that the end had come, or opportunities to intentionally conclude a life. While there were many disadvantages to these kinds of deaths, there was also a convenient clarity:

there was very little gray area between life and death (Fishman 2010: 67).

By contrast, prolonged dying processes make death's approach more complex. The ambiguity of what constitutes the beginning of dying, or the approach of death, can also be accompanied by social, emotional, and spiritual ambiguity. Gradual death allows the dying person to ponder his or her approaching mortality. As Stephen Kiernan explains, prolonged dying also offers choices that were previously unavailable.

> Death by degrees does mean that dying is different. It takes months, not minutes. For a rapidly growing number of people, dying has become a process. . . . When dying is a process, the manner and meaning of a person's final days are not left wholly to chance. There are options and opportunities; there are choices. (Kiernan 2006: 13)

Many of those choices are positive ones—the opportunity to intentionally conclude one's life, to say good-bye to loved ones, to take a final trip, and to communicate one's wishes. Some choices are much more challenging, including how to manage the caregiving required by slow decline and increasing dependency, how to pay for the extended expenses that accompany the final stages of life, and how to live a meaningful longer life.

The dilemmas of the threshold arise in part because new technologies make possible longer lives but do not instruct how to morally and ethically apply those technologies. How do we know it is time to quit trying to elongate life and live with the moments, hours, or days that remain? How old is old enough? For example, one of the family caregivers I interviewed, a woman named Janet Conroy, took care of her mother first at home and then as she moved into a CCRC. She describes what she calls the "roller coaster" she and her mother rode together while trying to make sense of their experiences. When I asked her what she would now tell a family caregiver whose loved one had just been diagnosed with a terminal illness, she said, "I would tell them to expect a bumpy ride."

> Expect it to feel like a roller coaster. Even though you think you can get everything figured out and straightened out, that might happen for a while, but something will shift, something will change. You'll have another thing to deal with. Just expect it to be a road full of challenges unlike what you've seen before. Try to let yourself shift with the person. Don't think of them as the same. Mourn your loss now, because they've changed. So try to move on with them instead of trying to keep them where they were.

This caregiver developed ways to cope with the many changes that characterized her mother's experience of the final stage of her life. When living in the threshold, many individuals struggle to know when the line between living and beginning to die has been crossed. The person diagnosed with the illness and his or her circle of support all want to know: how long do we have? Is this active dying?

The ambiguity of prolonged dying forces a series of difficult decisions that the dying and their loved ones, sometimes with the help of experts, must make. As scholar Mary Pipher points out, such decisions are often complicated by the lack of social support and lived experience that might make individuals more confident in how to proceed. "From both generations I hear stories of conflict, frustration, guilt, and anger. Meanwhile the old often feel unappreciated, stressed, and guilty. Hurt feelings often come from taking *personally* problems that are cultural or developmental. As a nation, we are not organized in a way that makes aging easy"

(1999: 7). Pipher worries that without a sense of the broader context for how we die now, individuals will experience greater shame and grief regarding their choices and actions during the threshold period between simply aging and actively dying.

How we die now challenges our ability to care for our loved ones with integrity and with confidence. The sudden deaths that were more common in the past gave way to the immediate expression of grief. Now, our advanced brains have produced preventive measures and new technologies that present us with a kind of ending that has no obvious response to accompany it. What's more, these longer endings open up possibilities for intervention that were unavailable to other animals, or to earlier humans. Writing about animal grief, journalist Diane Ackerman explains some habits of expression we can witness in other species.

> A 2005 study of elephant grief, reported in the Royal Society journal *Biology Letters,* confirmed what experts have long sworn, that elephants pay homage to their fallen, visiting the remains of even long-dead relatives, and gently turning over the bleached bones with trunk or foot. Biologists tell of gorillas banging their chests with yowls of anguish during a wake for a fallen friend, of sea lions wailing when their babies have been mutilated by killer whales, of grief-stricken monkey mothers carrying dead infants around for days, of geese singing both halves of a duet when their partners have died. (2011: SR9)

In the past, humans could mourn like other animals. Now that our dying is slower, more anticipated, and more controlled, we no longer have obvious rituals to accompany our grief. We may grieve the elongation of life, not just the end. We might even grieve the decisions we make in the longer window provided by the threshold. It's one thing to miss our loved ones who die before us. It's an entirely different feeling to believe we have let them down, prolonged their pain, or failed them.

Medical technologies create new confusions, including the mistaken perception that death itself can now be controlled. A physician interviewed for the PBS *Frontline* documentary "Facing Death" described how medical technologies increase confidence while complicating decision making.

> The uncertainty is the most disturbing part of the decision making, and the availability of the therapies has created this fiction that we can orchestrate this one way or another when the truth of it is that for all this magnificent technology, the underlying illness and the medical condition of the patient are far and away the most important factors in determining the outcome. But it feels like when you have the medical technology available that your decision to use or not use it is like the decision to allow life or not allow life, and that's not a position anyone wants to be in. (2010)

Unlike the animals that Diane Ackerman describes, contemporary humans are surrounded by the illusion of control. Increased longevity is itself partially the product of advances in medical technology, yet those same technologies do not allow one to predict how or when death will come.

Like the "fiction that we can orchestrate" that the physician refers to, the dying process also leads dying individuals and their loved ones to think they should be able to exert more control than they actually can. One woman I interviewed, who did not want to be named, still mourned years later that she had not used the technology at her disposal to *hasten* her loved one's decline when the possibility of meaningful existence had diminished.

I don't know how careful I should be about saying things, but some of us thought the process should be a little more . . . allowed to happen naturally in its own time, but some of us thought that we should maybe step up the medication a little bit. Um, some of us felt that she was in pain and wanted more medication, and some of us thought that what we were seeing and hearing from her was just more of the natural process of dying, so, you know, I think that . . . the hospice nurses weren't there 24/7. They would kind of check in on you, but other than that you're kind of on your own. It was hard, I think, to mitigate that, especially toward the end, so that's sort of a challenge that I remember.

This woman struggled beneath the burden of choice, whether or not she should use her access to painkillers to hasten her mother's end. The choice she made still rests heavily on her conscience. Even when families reconcile themselves to the likely outcome of death, they do not always know how long the disease will take nor can they anticipate the particular path the disease will take. Caregivers, the dying themselves, and medical experts all try to adapt to rapidly changing conditions within a longer dying trajectory.

Longer lives carry with them more days and hours to pursue life's pleasures, to show affection to the people we love, to make contributions to our communities, and to reconcile the meaning of our life and mortality. On the flip side, slower declines create new dilemmas. The longevity dividend produces a whole new chapter of life. That chapter comes at the end of life, when individuals are more likely to struggle with physical or cognitive disabilities. Longer lives are accompanied by different ailments, particularly the likelihood of multiple disabilities and dementia. The longer one lives, the more likely one is to suffer from multiple chronic conditions, particularly Alzheimer's disease. The chance of developing Alzheimer's disease *doubles* every year after the age of sixty-five. By the age of eighty-five, *one in two* people suffers from the disease (Fishman 2010: 133). Even if elders evade dementia and successfully navigate a social environment that was not built with their needs in mind, they often outlive their social network, surviving the deaths of spouses, friends, and even children and grandchildren. These changes have consequences for interactions within families, neighborhoods, and communities.

The dilemmas of the threshold are accompanied by a whole spectrum of fears and concerns. Caregivers—both paid and unpaid—worry that they will let down the dying persons, deprive them of time to live, diminish the quality of their days, run out of financial support, run out of compassion, or borrow the energy they need to care for elders from other important work, like caring for one's self, making a living, or caring for other dependents. Elders also worry as a result of the longer window of time and the decisions the threshold affords. Elders are concerned most about being a burden and about being in pain. They are also troubled about finances, outliving their loved ones, being neglected, and, finally, living a lonely life (Brabant 2003). These dilemmas take place within a dominant culture that largely avoids the subjects of aging and dying.

The American Way of Aging

American society is made up of many overlapping cultures and subcultures based on race and ethnicity, region, class, faith, values, and history. Within this mix, families and communities vary with regard to their beliefs, rituals, and practices concerning intergenerational rights and responsibilities. Despite these variations, some characteristics of the nation itself, and particularly of the relationship between the state and its people, distinguish an "American" approach to aging. First, as with other needs, Americans are much more likely than people of other nations to seek out paid help for themselves and their loved ones. Over the last sixty years as the number of nursing homes has increased, the tendency in the United States has been to treat the needs for elder care and support (much like the need for child care) as a private matter, to be negotiated by individual families and with the services provided by the private, for-pay marketplace (Abel and Nelson 1990). Americans have sought solutions to the elder boom not in communities, neighborhoods, or even extended family networks, but rather in home services, nursing homes, and CCRCs to serve the needs of elders as they age and require more assistance. In some nations, making a profit from caring for the dying and the aged would be viewed as profane, but not in the United States, where nearly 70 percent of elder care facilities are for profit.

While citizens of other nations look to the state to support their needs, many Americans demonstrate a fear of big government and the expansion of social services, no matter how deep the need. The most recent evidence of this distrust of government and trust of the marketplace is the fierce opposition to "Obamacare," which many politically right organizations describe as limiting their freedom. For conservatives, the notion that health care is a collective concern is abhorrent (Brown 2004). Regarding care at the end of life, one particularly American invention is for-profit hospice companies. In other nation-states, and particularly in England, where hospice originated, hospice is a state-provided service that is available to all citizens. When the government provides care, one result is that it is consistent across regions. In the United States, the reliance on market-based care means that the availability and quality of care are uneven as a result of location and the mix of nonprofit and for-profit services.

In addition to this market-based approach, several qualities associated with American history and beliefs actually work actively against a smooth transition to an older culture. First, the United States is a young country in terms of history, and it is a country that embraces youth and shies away from aging. Mary Pipher argues that "aging in America is harder than it needs to be" (1999: 16) because many Americans hold death at a distance and, as such, are inexperienced in dealing with mortality. This distance also makes discussions of how to cope with cultural change stilted if not impossible. As Kerry Egan points out, "For reasons both cynical and clinical, the American political debate on health care treats end of life care like a contagion—an unspeakable one at that" (2012). Anyone who witnessed the national debate on what came to be known as death panels in 2010 can testify to the sort of hysteria that can accompany frank discussion of changing end-of-life conditions. As Americans grow older, the United States falls increasingly behind other nations in its willingness to discuss policies that address the demographic shift under way. Rather than sober deliberation, avoidance punctuated by occasional hysteria prevails.

The American approach to aging is currently characterized by four weaknesses. First, for all the potential advantages of institutionalizing elder care—a subject that this book will cover in depth—nursing homes currently segregate elders from the larger community. Too often, fears about vulnerability, dependency, and frailty are displaced and transformed into contempt for the elderly themselves (Fishman 2010: 289). Unfortunately, fostering fears about dependency and segregating elders do nothing to stem the tide of aging or the inevitability of mortality. Avoiding the many issues raised by living in a graying society only increases the possibility that the longevity dividend will be squandered, either individually or collectively.

Second, despite the systems for managing death—funeral homes, nursing homes, hospitals, mortuaries, and grief services—

death still poses a challenge in American cultures because it defies rationalization. Rationalization is the process associated with industrialization in which various aspects of life become increasingly subject to the principles of scientific management. Over time, as countries industrialize, systems develop to regularize aspects of everyday life, including eating, learning, healing, and even dying. The family is removed as the seat of social life, and social life is separated and rationalized into hospitals, day cares, therapists, elder homes, funeral homes, and so on. As it relates to old age and dying, industrialization also tends to make individuals less familiar with death and dying and to diminish the accumulated knowledge of elders.

Industrialization produces death novices because it separates individuals from the realities of death. Kiernan traces evidence of how "distant death has become" (2006: 51).

> For virtually all of human history people experienced dying at close range. They watched it occur, participated in preparing the body, constructed the coffin, dug the grave or built the pyre. If a person performed these tasks today, far from being perceived as devoted, he or she might well be considered ghoulish. Touching the corpse, even of a beloved, is taboo. A dead body is so alien in contemporary America that few people outside the medical field know what to do when they encounter one. From this unintentional ignorance, it is a long journey to treating a dying person with reverence. (2006: 51)

Dying is at once alien to many young people and inherently unmanageable. Despite illusions of control, the specific moment and conditions of dying are nearly impossible to fully control.

Beyond denial, it could be that Americans struggle with
death because they have made nearly everything else in
their lives subject to reason, systemization, and control—
from the timing of conception and manner of birth onward.
Only death remains outside the corral, the wild horse that
will not be tamed. (Kiernan 2006: 67)

This lack of control can be particularly difficult for individuals
who are used to living in carefully managed social environments.

Third, the ethos that accompanies American capitalism sets up
a system of values and rewards that diminish the significance of
the experiences of elders. American capitalism rewards productivity as an almost unquestioned good. Within capitalism, economic
productivity is the ultimate measure of value. When elders can
no longer participate in the marketplace as workers, their value
is diminished. As Phyllis Star, one of the chaplains I interviewed,
explains, "Many people don't know what to do in the latter years
of their life, when they're not taking their identity from work, and
that's gonna be crucial because people are going to have thirty
years of their time there." While in "traditional" societies, elders
are sought out for advice and assistance, in postindustrial societies,
older adults are less often honored or esteemed because traditional
knowledge is replaced by the expertise of specialists associated with
rationalization (Crampton 2009). The conditions of global capitalism have also influenced intergenerational connections as extended
families are spread farther across the country and the world, "creating a transient class less tethered to older relatives for practical
and emotional support" (Fishman 2010: 288). The more elders live
alone rather than with family, the more distance there is between
elders and members of younger generations, deepening the intergenerational divide.

Finally, alongside capitalism, the relentless pace of new technologies often diminishes the importance of elders' skills and knowledge. New technologies can make older ways of doing things seem or become obsolete. Many elders find themselves struggling to live in a world that has used technology to increase the speed and complexity of daily life. Elders navigate a landscape that is primarily set up for able-bodied young people in a society that has yet to build the infrastructure to accommodate the needs of a much older population. Elders deal with fast highways; oversized, crowded consumer outlets; complicated travel centers; small-print books, brochures, and menus; dark and loud public venues; and steps, stairs, and uneven terrain throughout their days. The unforgiving landscape is reinforced by depictions of elders in popular culture. Popular culture celebrates youth and generally presents elders as unimportant, dependent, or sources of comedy. Realistic representations of the complexity of old age are incredibly rare. The celebration of youth and the virtual silence around old age carry incredible social costs: they prevent us from living the longevity dividend intentionally and from making more of and fearing less the features of prolonged dying. As Mary Pipher writes, "Bodies last longer than brains, support systems, or savings accounts. We don't have the resources, the rituals, or the institutions to make our old feel like elders" (1999: 17). Taken together, these tendencies, some of which crosscut American cultures, and some of which characterize only pockets of American life, all shape attitudes about old age, quality of life for elders, and interactions between generations.

Old-Age Institutions

In the United States, the conditions of societal aging bring Americans into contact with an often dreaded and feared social institution: the nursing home. According to recent studies, as many as 70 percent of Americans wish to end their lives in their own homes, but only 30 percent of them manage to die in the way they prefer (Brabant 2003). Given the prevalence of this experience and the significance of institutions in the final years, understanding the interactions that characterize these institutions and gaining insight into how these institutions support, sustain, and even innovate under new social conditions is particularly important.

Many Americans who have an opportunity to experience the longevity dividend will spend some of their days, months, and years in an elder care facility. In 2012, the elder care industry as a whole comprised 16,100 nursing homes with 1.7 million beds (Centers for Disease Control and Prevention 2011). At more advanced ages the chances of living in a nursing home rise steeply: in 2008, only 7.1 percent of the elderly resided in nursing homes, but among those eighty-five and over, the proportion increased to 11 percent, and among those over ninety-five years of age, that number rose to 38 percent (National Institute on Aging 2011; U.S. Bureau of the Census 2009). Although the majority of Americans wish to die at home, 43 percent of all Americans over sixty-five will spend at least some time in a nursing home during their lives, and 70 percent of Americans will die in either an elder care facility or a hospital (Kiernan 2006: 10).

Elder care institutions care for elderly people while also producing and responding to ideas, attitudes, and fears regarding old age and death. Longer lives have produced high levels of disease acuity. Acuity measures the severity of an illness and the attendant need for care. While some elders will live longer, they are living longer precisely because medical technology has allowed them to survive diseases that would have killed them in previous generations, and as a result, their bodies are often compromised by the traces of previous diseases and disorders. Like other changes associated with societal aging, these changes are not at all slow but, rather, dramatic. Elder care facilities have adjusted to changing needs by building larger memory units for the care of residents with Alzheimer's disease, expanding dining rooms to satisfy baby boomers' aesthetics and to make space for the greater proportion of wheelchair users, and increasing staff to assist with feeding and bathing residents at home and in assisted living. Not only have elder care facilities changed considerably from their original form, but so have the life courses, acuity levels, and needs of the people who live within them.

This book is designed to move the reader through and beyond the many fears that attend the social conditions of old age to a renewed sense of hope as we witness the connections that bind us to one another to the end of our days. Because of how old age is currently structured, the outstanding opportunity of the longevity dividend may at times appear to be a social problem. But the social problem is not our longer lives and slower deaths; the problem is our lack of a language and a series of practices that will help us experience longevity in ways that are fulfilling and expanding for participants. This is not to say that no one in our midst has figured out how to navigate the new social terrain of old age. Rather, that knowledge and experience are not shared as they might be: they get caught or trapped in the memories of individual families who have helped their loved ones die and, more specifically, they are housed in the minds and understanding of workers who routinely help others navigate the waters of old age and dying. In what follows, I challenge readers to think about the possible role of institutions in these developments. Is it possible for dying to combine professional expertise with familial support? I argue that we need to have open minds as we seek the wisdom to make the last years of life manageable: some will turn to religion, others to medicine, and some to a host of other professionals—social workers, nurses, nurse's aides, and hospice workers—who have made this stage of life the subject of their paid employment.

Right now in the United States, we want to age well; we just have not decided how to do that within the limits of our bodies and the context of our culture. Doing death differently is an opportunity. We need not long for a time when accidents and unmitigated diseases killed us quickly, or when old age was a rarity rather than a likelihood, or for a time when gender regimes required women to provide unpaid care to the aged and dying at home. None of these reversals is likely to occur, nor does it need to in order to find our way through to not just dying but also living differently. In this book I intend to convey the clarity and confidence that elder care workers already possess. I argue that our approach to death could be improved if we seize on what these workers know.

Studying the End of Life

The stories and findings I convey here are drawn from over fifty interviews with chaplains, social workers, physicians, certified nurse's aides (CNAs), nurses, residents, and administrators. Interviews were semistructured, meaning that I went in with about twenty questions but also followed up on stories and insights from each participant. Each interview lasted from twenty minutes to three hours. Potential interviewees were invited to participate using the snowball sampling technique, in which the first participant recommends or refers additional voluntary participants. The snowball sampling technique uses existing social and occupational networks to reach a growing number of participants over time. The majority of these participants were living or working in the primary research site, Winthrop House, while the rest worked or lived in nearby facilities.

To provide some context for the interview data, I also spent several years observing everyday activities at Winthrop House. First, in 2008, I completed seventy hours of training and passed the exam to become a certified nurse's aide (CNA). Next, I completed clinical training at Winthrop House as a CNA. My participation in CNA training was designed to familiarize me with the rules and regulations governing contact and interactions with residents in long-term care facilities. I also trained as a hospice volunteer with the hospital that provides hospice support to Winthrop House. Between 2009 and 2012, I then spent over two hundred hours observing everyday activities at Winthrop House. I sat in on administrative meetings, attended regional conferences, had lunch with residents, volunteered with the activities department, visited residents in hospice, and attended gatherings in order to draw some conclusions about how Winthrop House residents and staff interact, communicate, and connect.

Ongoing, unfettered access to Winthrop House has allowed me to follow up on hunches, observe bedside interactions, and continually build the network of participants in this study. While the remarkable support and cooperation of Winthrop House have provided a home base for those inquiries, this study is not place-specific but rather is categorical in its focus. I wanted to hold place constant, to study what this one place might tell us about how we arrange aging and dying, the fears that surround these experiences—both founded and unfounded—and the human dilemmas that arise and are confronted through interactions at the end of life. So what begins with one institution provides a vantage point on how we age and die now.

This project makes use of one facility in a small midwestern town as a laboratory to research the interactions among workers, residents, and their families as they negotiate needs, time, expert knowledge, and care at the end of life. It is specifically about old age and dying: my research does not address deaths earlier in life; rather, it addresses the whole range of wellness, fitness, disability, and disease that can accompany old age. The participants in this study are gathered by virtue of the fact that they live or work in a CCRC. Some of the residents are well elders, while others are actively dying. Studying a CCRC allows me to study individuals in a range of health states, including the same individuals as they move across a range of services and situations within the same CCRC: from independent living, to assisted living, and into full-time nursing care.

Both of these processes—elongated lives and prolonged dying processes—take place within the ten square blocks that make up Winthrop House. Although much about American culture would have us believe that dying is scary and unpredictable, for the workers who aid their residents during their final chapters, death is no longer scary or unpredictable. Paid caregivers help elderly and dying residents and their loved ones recognize what is *common* in our aging and dying processes. Workers use the knowledge that they derive from daily engagements with mortality to help residents recognize important signposts in the final chapter of life. Meanwhile, residents and their family members are actively engaged in making sense of their own changes within the larger social context of longer lives and slower dying processes. Combining the voices and insights of workers, residents, and administrators allows me to convey the lessons from the end of life that each group of participants has mastered.

Located in a midwestern state with high rates of longevity, Winthrop House is in a town that I call Littleton, one that provides a particularly good site for staging such a study because it is regarded as a "good place to die" by townspeople and is known as a place with high-quality end-of-life services. Littleton is a small, socioeconomically diverse town of just under ten thousand people, with a high density of residents over the age of sixty-five. With a small college as one of the more prominent organizations in town, Littleton is a destination for college students; it is also a place where many people return to retire. In recent years, as baby boomers have begun to retire, college towns have become popular places for retirees in the United States and Canada to settle (Fishman 2010: 234) because they offer free or reduced courses to elders; provide substantial free arts, sports, and educational programming; and offer a way for new residents to become engaged in the local community. Littleton is a face-to-face community, meaning that service providers and recipients are often known to each other prior to their connections within service interactions. The stories from Winthrop House provide an "in the trenches" look at social change as it happens in one specific town in the Midwest.

Case studies that focus on a particular place or group of people in extensive detail have much to offer us because ethnographic studies provide a kind of familiarity that goes beyond summary and gets to the nuance of human experience (Geertz 2000). The *advantage* of doing an in-depth study of one specific site for old age and dying is that this approach allows me to know one place well and to convey the stories and insights from that place to my readers. The *disadvantage* of this approach is that having only one case from which to draw conclusions can limit the generalizability of my findings and conclusions. Winthrop House is the product of a particular location in a particular region at a particular time in history. Much of what occurs there may be predictive of daily practice at other similar sites; however, much may be particular to the people who inhabit the space and the history and customs that inform their interactions. Nevertheless, I show that the residents and workers at Winthrop House provide windows into the conditions of living and working in an elder community. Participants in this study are pioneers in the social environment that now accompanies aging and dying processes, a terrain that has changed considerably over the past century and into which they offer insight.

The specific history and location of Winthrop House shape daily practice and affect who is drawn to live and work there. For example, certainly it matters that Winthrop House is a *not-for-profit* long-term care facility. As a CCRC, the Winthrop House provides shelter and staged levels of care for residents who are entirely independent all the way to residents who need around-the-clock care. So, while many people would casually refer to the place as a nursing home, it is not. Nursing homes are facilities that have spaces only for residents who need regular, daily medically certified care, while a CCRC offers twenty-four-hour medical care as one level of care in a much larger community of residents who are fifty-five years of age or older. All of this work is done with the goal of breaking even, not making a profit. It is also relevant that Winthrop House has been in business for more than half a century and has a reputation for providing excellent care and for having a wealthier clientele than the other two facilities located in the same town. (Although the realities of the economic privilege of the residents do not live up to this perception, as I explain in Chapter 2, this perception matters.) Located in a predominantly white state, in a predominantly white town, Winthrop House is *unlike* many elder care facilities in terms of its racial homogeneity. While in other locations racial minorities would make up a significant fraction of the residents and in many cases the majority of workers, by contrast, Winthrop House is more than 90 percent white. Studying a racially homogeneous CCRC might obscure some of the dynamics that influence everyday life in the majority of elder care facilities. Despite these limitations, I hope that this study illuminates tendencies in this stage of life that are true regardless of the racial makeup and dynamics of participants.

Lifting the Curtain on the End of Life

When I tell friends, colleagues, or family about the subject of my research, I often receive the now familiar reply "How depressing!" If you, too, are concerned that having cracked the cover of this book, you will be taken down a dark path into the unknown territory of old age, I want to offer an alternative perspective. Knowing about longer lives and prolonged dying processes is *empowering*—it gives us options and it wipes clear the shadows that so often shroud the final years and days of life. I think of the stories and experiences gathered here as offering a sociological handbook on how we age and die now, sort of like a *What to Expect When You're Expecting* but for the final years. Expecting death and knowing old age do not need to be depressing. That is what the people described in these pages taught me.

Over the last five years as I have journeyed further into the land of old age, I have been frequently surprised at how eager participants are to tell their stories: volunteering in the grocery line, asking for updates about my work, and sending photos and late-night e-mails about their own experiences and memories of assisting others in their final years, days, and hours. When I first began this research, I felt as though I had stumbled into a social wound—a space of unarticulated pain that was just looking for expression. But I was quickly corrected in that assumption; the stories that workers and residents were eager to tell were profound and often healing or beautiful rather than painful. Even when the interviewees had to pause several times to cry about memories, they were often insistent about sharing their stories of what someone else's end-of-life process had taught them about themselves, about dying, and about living. I hope the stories and experiences captured here prove to be a source of curiosity, comfort, and maybe even inspiration for readers.

We are aging and dying in ways that are *unlike* how our ancestors died, and we find ourselves ill prepared for what could potentially be a gift. My hope is that hearing from one community of individuals navigating the experiences of elongated life and prolonged dying might help demystify what Mary Pipher rightly calls the "unknown country" of old age (1999). For many of us, old age and the changes that accompany prolonged dying are truly "another country." I hope that this book brings that territory close at hand, allowing readers to explore the many challenges and fears that come with the new conditions of our final years and days, as well as the rewards and pleasures that longer lives can provide.

2

The Paradox of Long-Term Care

We Need It; We Fear It

One often-told story at Winthrop House is that in the late 1950s, two lively female residents—Martha Breman and Barbara Weck—were flying back from a trip to Australia at the same time that the *Sputnik* rocket was returning into earth's atmosphere. According to the story, Martha said, "What if *Sputnik* hits our plane?" and Barbara replied, "Well, at least we won't have to move to the care center!" Like Martha and Barbara, many if not *most* Americans dread the "final move" to a nursing facility. Some might even rather die in an explosion to avoid a slow fading away in a nursing home bed. At Winthrop House, this fear is embodied in the move to the care center, the part of the continuing care retirement community (CCRC) that has twenty-four-hour nursing and is therefore associated with dependency and finality. For most Americans, the fear of the final move is more diffuse; it attaches not onto a specific place but rather onto *all* the spaces associated with end-of-life care. In fact, I argue that all the fears that surround the end of life—needing assistance, losing control, losing one's individuality, becoming totally dependent, being neglected—often get attached to a specific institution: the nursing home.

There are also many concerns about living longer lives without the kind of structural and social support that might make longer durations of dependency less frightening. The longevity dividend delivers more years that raise a host of concerns worth worrying about: becoming a burden to relatives, losing life savings to end-of-life care, and running out of options for support as bodies and minds change and succumb to multiple conditions. While many of these fears are actually about longevity, ability, and independence, these fears tend to be directed, somewhat irrationally, at the one institution that attempts to provide for systematic elder care: the nursing home. I argue that those fears are outdated and costly. Latent critiques of the (lack of) public policy and social structure are deferred by attention to the faults and downfalls of institutionalized elder care. Perhaps most importantly, fear can be paralyzing—it can delay decisions at the end of life, and it can prevent individuals from reaching out to those who have developed expertise about how we age and die now. In this chapter, I explore the beginnings of elder care facilities and the origins of the fears that continue to plague these institutions. I discuss how the fears that attach to these places are really fears about old age itself that can be addressed once they are acknowledged. Finally, I reveal how these fears operate like a veil that prevents a more sober and intentional approach to old age.

Elder Care Facilities: Why We Need Them

Although the vast majority of Americans report a desire to die at home, less than half do. In a recent Time/CNN poll, 70 percent of those questioned wanted to die at home, but in reality, 75 percent of Americans die in hospitals, fighting death with all the available medical technology, or in nursing homes, after changes in health make it impossible to remain at home (Brabant 2003). American elders do not want to live in nursing homes. For example, in a survey of three thousand seriously ill hospitalized patients, "25 percent said they were unwilling to and 30 percent said they would rather die than live in a nursing home—only 2 percent said they would do so voluntarily" (Olson 2003: 104). Despite the fear and dread such places inspire, because we are living longer and dying slower, more Americans will spend part of their lives in elder care facilities. One million Americans move into a residential care facility every year. In fact, 2 percent of all elderly people reside in an elder care facility. For those who live to eighty-five years of age, the percentage residing in elder care rises to 25 percent. Forty-three percent of all older people eventually will spend at least some time in a nursing home (Olson 2003: 108). So the paradox of long-term care continues.

As longevity expands, the duration of old age expands disproportionately. There is an often asked question—meant to spur debate and reflection—that goes something like this: If you could live forever, what age would you want to be? With the longevity dividend, the extra years of life come in the seventh, eighth, or ninth decade. As a result, the longevity dividend means being older for longer. Of that extra thirty years that many people born in the twentieth century get to enjoy, many of the years involve increasing levels of disability that make the activities of daily living (ADLs) challenging, if not impossible, without the assistance of a paid or unpaid caregiver. ADLs include eating, bathing, grooming, dressing, walking, toileting, and getting in and out of bed or on and off chairs, while *instrumental* activities of daily living (IADLs) include housekeeping, laundry, and other maintenance chores; shopping; food preparation; managing money; and paying bills. Many elders need help with both, and in the absence of a reliable system for in-home care, many elders reach a point in their lives when it is no longer safe for them to attempt to live alone or with their partner at home.

Elongated lives, changing hospital patterns, and the incidence of dementia all contribute to a growing demand for elder care facilities. Depending on their ability level, freedom from chronic illness or pain, and mental acuity, many people in their sixties and seventies can continue to live independently. However, by the time Americans reach their eighties, the likelihood of needing sustained assistance grows substantially. Many elders first enter a nursing home for respite or recovery after being treated at a hospital, not yet well enough to return home or function independently. This is in part because changes in hospitalization patterns and regulations have resulted in an overall tendency to release patients "quicker and sicker" from hospitals. According to the Federal Interagency Forum of 2000, between 1990 and 1998 alone, the average length of a hospital stay was reduced from 8.8 to 6.1 days. Older patients are moved out of hospitals "'quicker and sicker' shifting significant responsibility for intensive medical care to nursing homes, home health agencies, and especially the elderly and their caregivers" (Olson 2003: 24). Hospitals respond to new mandates to release patients more quickly to curtail costs, which leads to many admissions to nursing homes each year. As a result, many elders are being released from the hospital with medical needs not easily met in the home setting.

Furthermore, while dementia has always been a driving force behind the need for round-the-clock institutional care, the increased incidence of Alzheimer's disease has contributed to a greater need and demand for nursing home care. Although many Americans are keenly aware of the changes in ability and identity related to Alzheimer's disease and other forms of dementia, news sources and public debates rarely grapple with the true rate of Alzheimer's disease. *One in ten* people will develop Alzheimer's disease in their lifetime. What that often-touted statistic does not capture is that the greatest risk factor for Alzheimer's disease is age. The likelihood of developing Alzheimer's disease *doubles* every five years after the age of sixty-five. After the age of eighty-five, the likelihood of living with Alzheimer's disease grows to a remarkable *1 in 2* (Alzheimer's Association 2010). Since there is no cure for Alzheimer's disease, the increased incidence of the disease is just beginning to reshape the needs of residents and their families and the practices of workers in elder care communities. Workers in nursing homes are well aware of the prevalence of this frightening disease because the rooms and hallways are increasingly inhabited by residents struggling with the condition. In some nursing homes, as many as half of all residents suffer from dementia-related conditions that make their care at home nearly impossible.

In the late stages of Alzheimer's disease and with other forms of dementia, care of an elder becomes more of a team job than a task for one individual. Unlike elders needing physical assistance with ADLs, elders living with the later stages of Alzheimer's disease experience quickly changing moods, loss of impulse control, and extreme agitation. As a result, they eventually may need constant supervision to remain safe. Often, families are unable to provide such constancy at home because it is not suited for care, because they lack time and energy, or because they cannot afford round-the-clock paid help. These families often find themselves turning, however reluctantly, to the services of a nursing home. As a society, the United States must grapple with the likely prevalence of Alzheimer's disease for many of us who will receive the benefit of the longevity dividend. Even those Americans who have plans for how to stay in their own or a family member's home as they age may find that the care regimens required over time are too demanding to manage with the help of family alone. In short, the specter of Alzheimer's disease makes nursing homes increasingly necessary.

The paradox of long-term care is this: we want to live longer, but we don't want to need help. But we do need help. The fact that many of us will live in a nursing home at some point in our lives brings us in touch with several cultural fears. Examining and dismantling these fears may be a crucial step toward a systematic, intentional approach to enjoying our longer lives and slower deaths.

The Short, Sordid History of Nursing Homes

Part of the cultural fear surrounding elder care facilities may arise because elder care facilities are relatively new institutions, having grown exponentially in the last one hundred years. Over that time, nursing homes, as they have come to be called, have been plagued, rightly or wrongly, by bad press and a series of exposés on and investigations into abuse and neglect. Additionally, despite the growing availability and use of elder care facilities over the last hundred years, most Americans have limited firsthand experience with or knowledge about these organizations, and they continue to view the whole prospect of institutionalizing old age with suspicion. These attitudes likely originated from the development of "nursing homes" from other types of facilities and a lack of awareness about the variety of elder care facilities available today.

In the last hundred years, motivated by need, opportunity, and policy changes, many organizations have emerged to care for elders. These elder care organizations are actually quite varied: some are for profit, and some are not; some adopt business efficiency practices to turn a profit, and others do not; some provide a community for residents, and others give very specific, concentrated help to residents who do not interact with one another. Elder care actually takes place in a range of facilities, from simple age-specific housing complexes with light nursing care available (normally called assisted living) to complete CCRCs that include everything from independent living to twenty-four-hour nursing care, allowing elders to age *within* the same facility—what the industry refers to as aging in place. However, in the cultural imagination, there's very little nuance—when Americans think of what scares them, they often think of a very specific place, and that place is a "nursing home."

As a generic term, *nursing home* often does not specify a type of facility or set of services; rather, it refers to a site that is feared. In this usage, nursing homes are places where many Americans imagine being turned into a number, controlled by the staff, and put at risk of losing their identity, control, and independence. They imagine these places as "turning out" elder care like any other product. When people talk about their fears of such places, they describe long, gray hallways with old people crying out. They imagine unfeeling, overworked, underskilled staff, and finally, they imagine an organizational logic focused on providing minimum care for maximum pay. There are, without question, a few places that may fulfill these fears; there are, however, many more places that do not fulfill these expectations. Yet the cultural fears pervade. So while the term *nursing home* should refer to only an elder care facility with twenty-four-hour nursing, in the popular imagination it is used to describe *any place* where elders live and are cared for. This tendency to generalize is unfortunate because it sustains fears and muddies the distinctions among the actual range of organizations that specialize in elder care.

In my discussion, I refer to elder care facilities as nursing homes when talking about the rise of such organizations and the fears that surround them, but my discussion here is meant to dislodge the assumption that elder care facilities are uniformly bad and sad. I hope to uncover some of the origins of the stigma and distrust that have attached to elder care facilities as a means of offering a more nuanced understanding of the options available.

Compared to other institutions such as schools, churches, and prisons, nursing homes are new and growing quickly. Before the nineteenth century, no age-restricted institutions existed for long-term care (Ekerdt 2002: 1005). Historically, care of the dying was kin work, provided most often by female family members. During the 1800s, an institutionalized system arose to care for indigents who had no next of kin to care for them. Over time, public houses and almshouses were created to care for poor elderly who could not provide for their own care (Ekerdt 2002: 1004). Part of the early stigma associated with nursing homes evolved because such houses often combined care of the elderly with care of any other members of society who could not manage by themselves, including severely disabled younger people and mentally ill citizens of all ages. By the turn of the twentieth century, the deplorable conditions of almshouses had garnered the attention of public reformers, and calls were made for better alternatives (Olson 2003: 158). Between 1900 and 1930, most of the alternatives were nonprofit facilities run by religious charitable organizations. Although these institutions have changed greatly in the last hundred years, nonprofit elder care facilities continue to share the originating philosophy of almshouses and poorhouses that caring for elders should *not* be associated with a profit. The early nursing homes were implicitly regarded as similar to other types of institutions that were founded to care for dependent adults, including asylums for the mentally ill and boarding homes. So even though nursing homes have changed a great deal, particularly since the 1980s, many people continue to imagine them as warehouses for the old. Many Americans have limited contact with elder care facilities and know little about the origin of such places. This unfamiliarity can breed suspicion.

Elder care facilities were not intentionally developed in the United States; instead, they were created in response to a series of policy changes. Contemporary elder care facilities are largely the result of the Social Security Act of 1935, which dispersed old-age assistance program payments to elders directly, allowing them to choose their site of service. The same act *disallowed* payments to public houses, thereby triggering a massive relocation of elders from almshouses to *private* boarding homes and nursing homes (Ekerdt 2002: 1006). In short, this 1935 act launched the development of contemporary elder care facilities, making the United States the country with the most private facilities of this type. The number of nursing home facilities grew rapidly after World War II.

The next major stimulus to the proliferation of nursing homes came in 1965, with the enactment of Medicare and Medicaid. As early as 1970, only five years after the legislation passed, 75 percent of all residents in nursing homes were supported by Medicaid (Vladeck 1980). This flow of public monies into nursing homes opened up greater avenues for profit while also sustaining the perception that nursing homes were places for poor elders. Cumulatively, these policy changes made nursing homes big business by opening up high profit margins in a new and rapidly growing industry, subsequently expanding a still-young institution practically overnight. For example, between 1960 and 1976, the number of nursing homes grew by 140 percent, the number of nursing home beds increased by 302 percent, and the revenues received by the industry rose 2,000 percent (Ekerdt 2002: 1005). Between the year that Medicare and Medicaid were enacted and today, the nursing home industry has expanded dramatically and adopted many of the practices of big business through mergers and the development of large chains.

The American approach to old age is uniquely reliant on for-profit institutions. No other nation has the same density of for-profit sites. Today, over 68 percent of all elder care facilities are for profit (Ekerdt 2002; Centers for Medicare and Medicaid Services 2010). While there are high-quality and low-quality types of both for-profit and not-for-profit facilities, the for-profit chains have garnered a great deal of public and journalistic attention, therefore contributing to the general distrust of elder care facilities. Studies of for-profit elder care facilities demonstrate some of the specific risks that attach to a for-profit arrangement. The organizations are incentivized to admit wealthier residents (Anders 1997). Since demand exceeds supply in many places, for-profit providers can also select the wealthier potential residents from their waiting lists. While no study has shown consistently worse treatment in for-profit versus not-for-profit facilities, many Americans have concerns about mixing care of dependent elders with the profit motive. Fears that should be specific to for-profit institutions are often quite diffuse, spreading easily to all elder care institutions, regardless of the profit arrangement. Those who build or run elder care facilities labor against a cultural imagination that is very negative toward the work that they do, and that cultural imagination continues to be fed by reporting that fuels worst-case fears.

Scandal and Regulation in Elder Care Facilities

During the short history of nursing homes, Americans have been audience to a steady stream of journalistic and scholarly exposés regarding the industry, particularly since its early expansion in the 1960s. Considering its relatively brief existence, the elder care (or "nursing home") industry has been scrutinized and regulated at an unprecedented pace and scope. Here, I trace sources for the concerns that plague the industry as well as some of the underlying anxieties that may fuel such concerns. As early as the 1970s, a congressional study deemed nursing homes "warehouses" for the old and "junkyards for the dying" (Foundation for the Aid of the Elderly 2012). As recently as 2001, a congressional study identified abuse in as many as one-third of all facilities (Waxman 2001).

Congressional studies have reacted to and also informed news stories on the industry. Television news and newspapers feature many stories of gruesome neglect and abuse. The abuses reported reflect all the vulnerabilities of old age: sexual abuse and touching; verbal abuse and vulgarity; neglect; overlooking the needs of residents; unacceptable waiting time for assistance; physical abuse; and inconsiderate, unhealthy, or even illegal care of elders. Headlines expose nursing homes that evict residents who are too costly, nursing homes that close with no warning, and unsustainable staff-to-resident ratios that leave minimally trained workers in charge of far too many dependent adults. In the last three years, leading newspapers, including the *New York Times,* the *Wall Street Journal,* the *Chicago Tribune,* and the *Minneapolis Star Tribune,* all featured stories about the inadequacies of elder care facilities. Some of this reporting unveiled serious shortcomings, such as the hiring of staff without the performance of criminal background checks, while other "charges" seemed designed to simply fuel suspicion, as in articles about the frequency of lawsuits against nursing homes without mention of how many of those suits were dismissed or lost. There is a healthy appetite for and ready supply of stories about the failures of nursing homes. Remembered directly or recalled by family members in attitudes toward elder care facilities, these reports of abuse and neglect are sometimes the only information that families have about elder care facilities prior to the need to enter one.

Journalistic and scholarly studies of elder care facilities have uncovered evidence of abuse and neglect that have eventually formed the impetus for new policy. Scandals inspire change, but the improvements are rarely reported. Negative press is often the *only* kind of press that nursing homes receive. The mainstream media rarely present stories about high quality of life, good relations, healthy elder living, positive improvements, or innovations. In short, nursing homes are institutions plagued by bad headlines with no counterweight. As Olson explains, legislative attention has tended to react to exposés and scandals.

> Government interest in the problems, for the most part, has been scandal driven, with short-term damage control as the major goal. The politics and policies related to the neglect and mistreatment of nursing home residents have been a vicious cycle of "new" revelations, government studies, congressional hearings, additional rules and regulations, poor enforcement, and more disclosures. (2003: 109)

When scandal produces only new regulations with no follow-through or support for best practice, the cycle of scandal-policy-pause leads to uneven care in the most regulated industry in the United States. Meanwhile, some industry leaders have voluntarily changed the care they provide to offer residents better quality of life. Referred to as "culture change" and dating from the 1980s through the present, significant changes in terms of both space and interactions have been instituted at many places like Winthrop House. These changes are transformative, but are not regulation driven, and almost never reported. Both the government and the general public are audience to occasional frenzies regarding the negatives of elder care facilities with virtually no counterbalance, while the more mundane, satisfying experience of residents in elder care facilities rarely, if ever, make headlines.

Not surprisingly, then, fears persist with regard to an industry that developed without any large-scale planning to address a population of care recipients who did not favor the arrangement and that has, since its inception, been haunted by scandals and public outcries about the low quality of care it provides. One of my concerns is that the public receives a one-sided view of life in an elder facility that discourages further investigation into later-life living options. The press coverage also produces a stigma that influences how elders who are currently living in institutionalized care feel about their "home." Finally, media and policy attention has led to an exhaustive list of regulations that have done little to improve quality of life for residents across the board. In the absence of a systemic response to these criticisms, old fears are resilient and are even passed down between generations.

Unfortunately, left unattended, widespread public fear will not prevent individuals from needing or eventually succumbing to institutionalized care. Along with others, I worry that fears about nursing homes not only are largely misplaced but also get in the way of intentional decision making at the end of life. Fears prevent families and would-be residents from planning in advance and exploring the differences between institutions of varying quality, safety, and satisfaction. A more nuanced evaluation of nursing homes would reveal a whole range of services and quality. In what follows, I discuss two of the most prominent fears that plague institutional care.

Fear One: Places for the Unloved

The primary fear that seems to haunt nursing homes is that institutionalized elder care is substandard care for individuals who are not loved enough by their families to be cared for at home. In this view, nursing homes are locations for compensatory care—care that makes up for the care that families are unable or unwilling to provide at home. This fear and the guilt that accompanies it are so strong that they even cause residents and family members to distrust the caregivers in institutional settings. Elder care workers report such mistrust also stigmatizes their work: friends and colleagues assume that they had no other occupational options, that they are not smart enough to do other medical or social service work, or that they take care of elders because it is easy. Meanwhile, respondents to opinion polls in the United States imagine nursing homes as places of neglect and mistreatment. For example, in a national opinion poll in 2005, 53 percent of those surveyed believed that some nurse's aides abuse elders, 9 percent believed many abuse elders, and 5 percent believed all nurse's aides abuse elders (Kaiser Family Foundation 2005).

When fears about growing older and about institutionalized care become solely associated with nursing homes, they also free up other forms of end-of-life care from suspicion and shame. Elder care facilities are positioned in contrast to the safe, secure, even ideal care provided at home. An often unspoken but powerful assumption that drives the old-age paradox is that in-home care is automatically—even intrinsically—superior to institutional care. This belief protects care at home from scrutiny. However, while most Americans like to think about the dangers of home care even *less* than the dangers of institutional care, intentional and unintentional abuse and neglect also take place at home. Caregivers find themselves overwhelmed, underskilled, and underfunded to provide the kind of complete care they would like for loved ones.

One of the contributing factors to elder abuse and neglect at home is that expectations about family obligations have not been updated to address the longevity dividend (Logue 1991). Traditional beliefs that care of the elderly should be solely the responsibility of family members are based on different lifelines and dying trajectories. As Xiaomei Pei, director of the Gerontology Center at Beijing's Tsinghua University points out, even in countries such as China that insist on maintaining a traditional commitment to care of elders in multigenerational home care settings, this cultural expectation, if not mandate, was based on the duration of life in earlier eras.

> While Chinese people are quick to say that caring for elders is part of their cultural and religious tradition reaching back centuries, they conveniently forget that over most of their history, the traditions were practiced when the average life expectancy in China was no more than thirty-five. The demands on pious children were much lighter then. When parents got sick, their illnesses tended not to linger. They, like everyone on the globe before the advent of modern medicine and public health, tended to be able one day, sick the next, dead shortly thereafter. (Fishman 2010: 307–308)

Changing demographics, including how long humans are living and how few children humans are having, are adding strain to the social contract. In China in particular, the one-child rule has produced a tiny generation that many scholars worry will not have enough labor power to support and sustain members of the elderly generation as they retire and live out longer lives.

Ultimately, positioning care at home as the ideal circumstance does not take into account that nursing home care is often consistent with or superior to the care that can be provided at home. In reality, institutional elder care is not compensatory; it is different. It is for pay, skilled, intimate, but less so than care by the family. It is heavily regulated, and it can be better than, worse than, or the same as care at home. Still, the belief that nursing home care is for people who are unloved persists.

One of the ironies of the compensatory care fear is that it may reduce involvement of family members when an elder does decide to enter or is placed in institutional care. Family members may fail to recognize the opportunity to partner with nursing home staff in caring for their loved ones, or they may let their own guilt about "having to rely on" institutional care prevent them from taking an active role in their loved one's ongoing care. As a response to guilt, family members may take themselves out of the care equation when an elder relative moves into institutional care. In so doing, they may perpetuate the very conditions for which institutional care is criticized: impersonal care by paid workers and isolation of elders from family. It is to this second major fear—that institutional care is invariably impersonal—that I now turn.

Fear Two: Institutional Care Is Impersonal

Another fear expressed by many Americans is that institutionalized elder care is depersonalized care that strips residents of their originality and individual identity. According to this concern, the move from private home space to shared, organizational space can represent the end of an individual self. Here the concern is that this "final move" marks the beginning of an unstoppable decline. Many elders fear that moving to a nursing facility means that they will no longer be able to sustain their abilities because the people who work in the institution will do more and more of the work of living for them until the elder becomes an invalid who is undifferentiated from the other resident patients.

This particular fear arises out of an intense focus on individuality that has old roots in much of American culture. In fact, individualism is so esteemed that any acknowledgment of dependency can be threatening. If one believes that dependency produces a loss of individuality, it is no wonder that some individuals fear elder care facilities. After all, elder care facilities are set up to respond to varying levels of dependency by facilitating activities of daily living so that residents become free to enjoy leisure, hobbies, and time with others. The move to an elder care facility also taps into concerns about dependency versus productivity. Under conditions of advanced industrialization, one's ability to be productive is highly valued. Living with assistance and living in a group environment both threaten the basis of an identity built on individualism and productivity. Like other fears, this fear has some validity to it: residents are often rewarded by staff for cooperating with care regimens, and a handful of residents do in fact fall into learned dependency patterns once they enter residential care. However, the move to an elder care facility need not mark the end of agency, direction, and unique personhood.

While there may be a handful of elder care facilities that deny elders their unique practices and preferences, vast improvements in elder care beginning in the 1980s through the present day— what is referred to as culture change in the nursing home industry—have made most of such places more like day cares or college dorms than not. This fear of being stripped of identity does not prevent elders from entering elder care, but it can shape how they approach their lives if they do move into a facility. The fear of depersonalization can be immobilizing for residents—it can cause them to keep to themselves, interact defensively with staff members, and fail to take part in the activities designed to build community among residents: games, rituals, celebrations, socials, performances, and governance groups. Particularly in assisted living and CCRCs, there is space for elders to pursue their own routines. Despite these conditions, the belief that life in elder care facilities is depersonalizing can itself cause harm. While elder care facilities certainly have an institutional logic that governs mealtimes and schedules, and regulations that dictate certain behaviors and limit others, many elder care facilities work hard to provide a homelike, community environment that allows residents to personalize their experiences, to continue to exert control over their days, and to pursue activities they enjoy.

Before they move to elder care facilities, many elders fear that institutionalized care will mean that they will be acted on like an object and treated like a number rather than a person. While there can be no question that institutionalized elder care makes use of group activities, daily routines, and timetables of activities that do not react to but rather organize residents' time, this generalized fear of conformity and being treated like others does not seem to adhere with equal forcefulness to other institutions that order the days of like-aged people. Schools and day care centers also group together age-mates for fun, learning, eating, sleeping, and sociability. Perhaps an accompanying fear here is that this particular setting—the nursing home—is not a training ground for other stages of life; it is the final institution to which most residents will belong. This apprehension about depersonalization is situated in a culture where old age is not uniformly valued. As such, the concern is that neglect or abuse is possible when one comes to be seen as simply "one of the old people." It might also reflect a belief that a place inhabited by elders will be uninteresting, depressing, or sad as compared to a place filled with children. When this fear is fed by scandals and stories of places that offer poor-quality care, it can be truly scary.

Do Not Lock Me Up in One of Those Places!

Mention that your loved one has entered a nursing home, and you are more likely to receive sympathy rather than support. Similarly, elder care workers are often pitied for "having" to work at a nursing home or CCRC. Many Americans even liken nursing homes to prisons. Like prisons and mental institutions, nursing homes are considered total institutions. "Total institution" is a concept developed by sociologist Erving Goffman to describe spaces where similarly situated people live together isolated from the larger culture and lead a formally ordered and managed life (1961). Nursing homes order the days and routines of the elders in their care. Elders' bodies are inspected, treated, and managed through institutional regimens. In these ways, nursing homes *are* like prisons. However, nursing homes are also a lot like schools, day cares, and college dormitories. Like-aged people are gathered, supervised, entertained, and protected from certain experiences for their own safety and protection. In fact, many elders who *enjoy* living in elder care facilities liken them to being back in college. What is it about elder care facilities as institutions that makes the more dramatic, more fear-inducing image of the prison the more common comparison?

I argue that fears about nursing homes combine mistrust of institutional life with more general concerns about aging. Fears about aging are primarily fears about declining autonomy. Many elders fear that as they age, they will lose a whole host of abilities that make them feel like fully human grown-ups who are in command of themselves. Features of autonomy include the ability to exert control over one's environment, to make choices, to reciprocate favors and gifts, to participate in daily life, and to pursue life's pleasures. So many of the fears that adhere to nursing homes are really fears about a time of life. Rather than honestly worrying about how we will manage old age, we redirect those anxieties onto institutions that house many people who are doing just that.

The specter of the nursing home hovers at the locus of our current old-age paradox: we fear the form of the help we need. Many of us want to age "gracefully," by which we mean living a long time with all of our abilities intact until we die one night in our sleep. We want to live longer, but we don't want to lose our capacities and abilities along the way. But that is not how the overwhelming majority of us will experience old age if we are lucky enough to live that long. We will, in fact, need help. When that help comes in the form of institutionalized care, another set of fears tends to combine with fears about autonomy.

This second set of fears is about our relationship to the marketplace. In short, distrust of nursing homes combines fears of dependency with more diffuse concerns about living in an advanced industrialized nation. In contemporary American culture, we move into and through institutions that "treat" us in one way or another. We move through institutions to be educated, to get married, to receive medicine, and to express our faith. Depending on our class status and what we can afford, we are also faced with an array of services from haircuts to massages, from gift wrapping to party planning, and from housecleaning to clutter consulting. These services have arisen because in the move away from the family economy, we have become specialists who rely on the services of others to fulfill many of our needs. In contrast to having the needs of individuals fulfilled by the expertise and labor of family members, industrialization breaks down all aspects of life into separate fields of action and expertise. Professionally, we train to do one thing. Consequently, we don't know how to do all the things we need to make life possible. Few of us know how to do all the tasks that would sustain a person: raise food, garden, cook, heal, teach, wash, weave, lift, build, create, and slaughter. Few of us are generalists; instead, we are specialists. Most of us are paid to do a narrow set of activities in our own working lives. We outsource many of our needs to experts in other fields; we do so more or less with ease, without alarm or moralistic debate. Most of us do not question whether or not we should go to the grocery store, yet many of us do struggle with how to negotiate the boundaries around services that we perceive as more intimate. So the emotions surrounding elder care facilities are in part about what we can trust institutions to do. Moving to or helping a loved one move to a nursing home raises the question: what kinds of activities are too intimate to pay for?

Turning over the care of elders to an institution inspires fear and shame because it touches on questions related to responsibility. Elder care facilities combine the logic of an institution with something precious and intimate—the care of elders. Often the person we, as family members, are helping to make the decision to move into a nursing home is someone who once took care of us: a parent, a spouse, or a friend. So it seems at times that *not* to return that care, or to put an end to that care, might be a breach of personal responsibility; it might violate one's obligation to loved ones.

Elder care institutions provide care that is at times intimate to individuals who are fragile and vulnerable. So the public worries, legitimately, about individuals or institutions that would abuse that vulnerability. A whole industry of watchdog groups and safeguards provides evidence of the prevalence of such worries. These safeguards include legal practices specializing in nursing home lawsuits, websites that track elder abuse, and elder monitors that are nearly identical to the devices parents use to monitor babysitters. Rather than "nanny cams" these are "granny cams." The websites that claim to track elder abuse share features with sites that claim to track pedophiles. Similar to abuse by strangers who prey on children, elder abuse is serious but rare. Children who are mistreated are usually abused by people at home whom they know. And so it is with elder care. Care in facilities is regulated and scrutinized far more than care at home, and workers are professionals—they are not motivated to hurt residents. Fears about vulnerability in old age get exaggerated and then directed at the particular site of the nursing home. These industries distract people into thinking that vigilance about nursing homes will protect against abuse. Unfortunately, what these watchdog industries cannot address are underlying concerns, and in some cases they seem to advance concerns.

The Costs of Our Fears

Persistent fears of nursing home facilities come at a cost. Whether based on fact, memory, or misinformation, fears about nursing homes shape family decision making about how to care for elders and policy and funding decisions about elder infrastructure. Sustaining these fears stymies more productive cultural debates about the proper care of elders. In short, even when we are faced with evidence to the contrary, fears about institutionalized aging and dying endure, preventing a more intentional approach to the development and regulation of elder care communities. My hope is that a close analysis of the myths and realities associated with nursing homes as institutions will invite a reappraisal that might move us closer to the sort of careful thought, debate, and commitments that are required to better meet the needs of a rapidly aging elder population.

At Winthrop House, activities staff struggle to get volunteers of any age to help with activities in the care center, the part of the facility that is perceived as a "nursing home." I asked about the residents who live in independent living: "Don't the people in the Winthrop apartments help out here? They volunteer with all kinds of organizations." The certified nursing assistant, Donita Mears, responded, "No, you'd think I would have dozens of volunteers, but they don't want to come over here [to the care center]. I think they're afraid. They don't want to see what is waiting for them." Like these would-be volunteers, many of us shield ourselves from environments connected to the end of life or death for as long as we can. Our fear of these places encourages us to stay away from others who are aging and dying. In fact, even among trained hospice volunteers in the United States, it is very difficult to find volunteers who are willing to go into nursing homes. So even those who volunteer their free time to help others at the moments of death avoid institutionalized sites of dying, preferring to help people die at home. I argue that cultural fears like those of the Winthrop House residents who refrain from helping their neighbors in the care center have detrimental effects. They are costly to the United States as a nation and to each of us as (hopefully) future elders.

First, because many Americans fear and distrust nursing homes, they often extend that suspicion to the individuals who work in nursing home settings and, as a result, fail to fully avail themselves of the workers as resources. In the United States, the work of caring for the dying is underpaid, poorly trained, and underappreciated. Consequently, the ability to stay removed from the end of life often functions along lines of privilege: the more privileged a person is in terms of social class, role in the family, gender, region, and race, the less likely one will be responsible for the care of a dying loved one. Privilege also shapes who does the for-pay care of individuals at the end of their lives. Across every region of the United States, the people who perform the frontline care of the elderly in long-term care facilities are those with few occupational choices; women, recent immigrants, racial minorities, and young, inexperienced workers all take care of the dying (Glenn 2010). The care of the dying is not honored as it might be—nor is it considered a calling, or an esteemed service to society, but it should be treated that way.

As a result of this low esteem, rather than reaching out to nursing home staff as experts on life changes in the final years of life, many residents and their families (at least initially) test and resist the help of staff. This is a waste of the kinds of assistance workers could and do provide to ease the transitions of the threshold. Attempts to care for loved ones through dramatic changes in needs and ability can be particularly difficult for family members who are encroaching on previously private terrain of their spouses, parents, or friends. As Mary Pipher explains, intimacy and respect for a loved one's privacy may prevent family members from asking the sorts of questions that are routine for workers.

> Out of a misguided respect for privacy, family members may not help one another enough. Adult children try to walk the fine line between being overbearing and neglectful. They may not ask, "Is someone abusing you?" "Do you need money?" "Are you taking the right amount of medication?" Their parents may not ask, "Do you think I'm losing my memory?" "Would you help me cut my toenails?" "Can I come with you?" (Pipher 1999: 123)

Elder care workers could partner with elders and their families to help anticipate changes and to set up systems that keep elders secure enough to live to the full extent of their limits, but often the resource of elder care workers is squandered.

Second, fears of nursing homes too often become justification for the disenfranchisement and categorical dismissal of elders more generally. In trying to forget these spaces for aging and dying, many people shield themselves from thinking about the group that largely inhabits nursing homes: elders over eighty-five years of age and anyone over sixty-five with significant cognitive impairments, particularly related to diseases like Alzheimer's disease. Such segregation and separation can deepen the distance between generations and perpetuate the lack of knowledge about the real effects of aging.

We isolate the end of life rather than embrace it, and our fears beget ignorance. As a result, the changes our bodies will predictably undergo are largely hidden, mysterious, and uncharted. Take the example of skin. As we age, our skin changes. Regardless of race, social class, or gender, our skin undergoes age-related change. Like baby's skin, elderly skin is distinctive: it tells its age; it is incredibly delicate, like tissue paper; it can tolerate very little soap because it is tender, like a baby's. However, unlike babies, we have almost no representations of what our skin will become if we live into old age. Elderly skin is beautiful, but we almost never see it represented in popular culture or in everyday life. As elderly skin becomes more common than baby's skin, shouldn't we have some sense of what to expect and how to care for this delicate skin as we do for that of our younger dependents? Skin is just one example of how age segregation leaves us uninformed and unprepared to care for ourselves and others in old age.

Third, fear accompanies less intentional responses to global aging and cultural change. The paradoxical circumstance in the United States is a fast-growing need for and diversification of elder care facilities amid persistent fear of the places. As a result, ideas about deservedness, familial obligations, and even changing gender norms all get attached to nursing homes and subsequently silenced. For example, focusing on how scary nursing homes are prevents discussion of why women—and particularly women of color—still provide the vast majority of care in the United States, even as women's participation in the labor force grows dramatically. It avoids a discussion of the stress on caregivers and the sometimes formidable costs—both material and emotional—of caring for loved ones at home. Nursing homes are places we do not talk about much, and as a result, we fail to critically engage with the social patterns that feed the paradox of expansion of nursing home care and persistent fear of that care.

Fourth, generalized fears about these places make it more likely that abuse and neglect will occur. Staff are overworked, underpaid, and underappreciated. While abuse remains rare, these labor conditions increase the possibility of neglect. Regulations abound, but few address or redress labor conditions that directly affect quality of life. Standards can be modified when knowledge and familiarity replace fear and avoidance. Rather than acknowledging the prevalence of nursing home care and working to consistently train workers, reward excellent workers, and fire bad workers, society, in its fear of nursing homes, also prevents against close scrutiny of the activities behind those doors and the vast differences between nursing homes. In fact, the general tendency in American culture to avoid death is costing us a lot on just about every level: individual, communal, and cultural. There is much to be learned about life at its end, but the majority of us do not know those things because we shy away, even run away if necessary, from the dying.

Setting aside fear and seeking knowledge and expertise are difficult because they require a frank acknowledgment of aging and shifting dependency. The changes that precede the move to a nursing home are anxiety-producing changes for both elders and their loved ones. Often, adult children and elder parents are shifting roles as adult children begin to take charge of their parents' care—a new and often uncomfortable change in power and authority. Mary Pipher captures some of the ways that everyone is off script, in uncharted terrain during these changes.

> Adult children are anxious about doing too much, and worried about doing too little. They fear parental disapproval or embarrassment, and they are nervous about making the wrong decisions at a time when decisions really matter. A bad call can mean death, squandered resources,

or lifelong regrets. Information isn't adequate, and every-body desperately wants to do the right thing. (1999: 122)

Harboring fear can get in the way of learning more about what to expect at the end of life and the available range of services. Questions about aging well, quality of life, anticipated duration of life, and the meaning of life often surface as elders experience changes in their physical and mental capacity. Making the decision to enter institutionalized care formalizes the need for assistance and may be the first shared acknowledgment of aging and a not-so-distant mortal end. Few families have a lot of experience with or knowledge of what institutionalized care entails, what they can expect, and how they should choose the best institution for their needs. Avoiding institutional care often means avoiding the help and expertise that might be crucial to an informed end-of-life experience. If we rest on these fears, we fail to have serious, difficult conversations that will have real, material consequences on decision making and quality of life in our later years.

Those who labor at the end of life have special knowledge about dying and about living, yet largely because of prevalent cultural fears, their knowledge often remains contained in the very institutions within which they work or within tight professional networks of communication and information sharing. Every industry has a few bad seeds—organizations that cut corners or abuse the trust of consumers. Unfortunately, the elder care industry has been reduced to memories and nightmares of a particular type of institution—the nursing home—which has few connections to the reality of daily life for elders living in a range of institutional care settings. Being assisted is the norm; abuse is not. Far from being places for the unloved, as the residents of Winthrop House attest, elder care facilities house elders with no families as well as elders with large, loving families, some of whom live right down the street. While a fraction of elders do decline, many blossom in their new living arrangement. In fact, some residents describe their time in an elder care facility as one of the best stages of their life. In Chapter 3, I move within the walls of a specific nursing home, Winthrop House, to examine how daily interactions there challenge many of the cultural fears about institutionalized aging and dying.

3

Transitioning Together

*Living, Working, Aging, and Dying
at Winthrop House*

A resident named Aida Dorenfield told me that at first she
was reluctant to move to Winthrop House with her husband. Now, three years later, she described it as the best
decision they have made. Aida described Winthrop House in the
following way:

> A warm, caring community "where life is added to years."
> A genuine retirement community, not an old folks home
> or a poor farm, much more than a "nursing home," though
> we have all those services (four levels of care, and a memory support unit with exceptionally good and caring staff).

Residents like Aida are aware of the many fears that surround
elder care facilities, but they believe that the place where they
live is special, desirable even. In explaining Winthrop House, she
alludes to less positive, even threatening ("poor farm"), images of
what collective living might be like. Residents also implicitly com-

pare life at Winthrop House with their previous lives in homes and apartments in age-diverse communities.

Like residents, Winthrop House staff members also labor against the reputation of elder care facilities as places that people simply move to in preparation for death. Staff members describe the dying process as only one small part of their interactions with residents during their time at Winthrop House. Instead, staff members are caught up in the challenges of providing a living context in which residents can lead high-quality lives. For example, a chaplain named Mary Montour who works at Winthrop House asks one of the philosophical questions that motivates her work: "So how do we re-create a sense of community when you're not living with your extended family? Your abilities are changing and you're dependent on people—how do you do that?" Like Mary Montour, staff and residents earnestly work to build and sustain a community within the ten square blocks of Winthrop House. They are proud of the relationships and quality of life they provide and enjoy.

In this chapter, I use the stories and experiences of Winthrop House residents to investigate the features and practices that make Winthrop House feel like a community to which one should move "sooner rather than later." My findings are based on survey responses from seventy residents. I asked them to explain why they moved to Winthrop House, the benefits and challenges of their lives there, the quality of their interactions with one another and staff members, any concerns they had at this stage, and what kind of plans (if any) they had put in place for their own end-of-life experiences. The survey tells a story of a group of empowered, deliberate, engaged citizens who range in age from fifty-eight to over one hundred years old. Residents' accounts upend expectations about what retired living is like, describing instead the benefits of a co-produced elder community. I then use observations from Winthrop House staff meetings to demonstrate what the trust and communication between staff and residents make possible as workers wrestle with the real challenges of aging and dying. I argue that, at its best, a close-knit environment like Winthrop House can assist residents in the transitions that accompany longer lives. I conclude the chapter by conveying stories *not* told, which reveal the implicit tensions between family care and institutional care.

Aida Dorenfield says that she would tell a friend that Winthrop House is an "eclectic group of folks with a general tolerance for diversity of beliefs, opinions, and habits," that this is a culture of "the glass half full," and that residents "have been and done all kinds of things, and most are still doing them." Aida is happy with her life at Winthrop House, and she is in good company. Amazingly, all seventy of the surveyed residents described a happy life at Winthrop House that suited their needs. They feel secure, they have good friends and neighbors, and they are confident in their surroundings. In fact, Aida was an outlier in that she took some convincing to move to Winthrop House. By contrast, many residents had long planned willingly to move there once they retired.

As Chapter 2 details, elder care facilities are places that are often feared and avoided. In this chapter, I use the voices and experiences of residents, nurses, chaplains, administrators, nurse's aides, and family members from Winthrop House to explore some of the challenges of building and sustaining an aged community. Their stories—both triumphant and challenging—disrupt common narratives about what elder care facilities are like and dislodge some of the more ubiquitous fears about elder care facilities. Like Aida, residents reflect a shared commitment to enjoy life. Some, like Aida, are won over; others choose Winthrop House for the positive mood of the place. Here, I use residents' own words to relate what facilitates a near consensus that Winthrop House is a good place to grow older.

Studying places like Winthrop House is essential as the United States moves toward being an aged society. Continuing care retirement communities (CCRCs) like Winthrop House become the staging ground for serious questions about how to survive old age and, ideally, how to live well in the later years of life. Who will care for us? Will we find pleasures amid changes in physical and cognitive abilities? Will we feel safe? Will our autonomy be the cost of that safety? These are the sorts of questions that residents and workers deliberate and determine through the day-to-day practice of living and working at Winthrop House.

Welcome to Winthrop House

As one of four elder care options in a small midwestern town of about ten thousand inhabitants, Winthrop House is known for its close connections to the local college and the quality of its in-house services, including grounds maintenance and food services. Winthrop House is affiliated with an elder care facility association called Leading Age, and Winthrop House administrators have held leadership positions at both that organization and faith-based organizations. While it is rooted in a faith tradition, it prides itself on a long history of providing a home for local citizens of all professions, faiths, and backgrounds. Residents range from retired ministers, college professors, and executives to retired farmers, housewives, and factory workers. One of the unique policies that residents and staff alike point to when they describe Winthrop House is that it promises a *permanent* home for residents. Unlike the vast majority of elder care facilities that may evict residents, Winthrop House has a need-blind policy specifying that once a potential client becomes a resident, he or she will never be asked to leave because of a lack of funding. In fact, in the history of the facility, no one has ever had to leave because of a lack of resources. This promise is sustained by a fund, which residents contribute to, that supports residents for whom the need arises.

In the town where it is located, Winthrop House is often referred to as the "fancier" of the elder care facilities. But despite this reputation, residents from a wide array of class backgrounds call the place home. While there are several rich residents, at any given time 40 percent of the current 260 residents are supported by Medicaid. In fact, Winthrop House works to correct the assumption that it is expensive to live there. While its costs are similar to those of the other facilities in town, the promise not to evict makes it potentially the most welcoming to less well-to-do residents. Despite these facts, the reputation of the facility, in part because of the close connection to the college, makes it seem upscale. This perception, then, shapes who considers living there and who does not. Residents describe this socioeconomic diversity as one of the best aspects of the place. They say that anyone can sit down at dinner with anyone else, regardless of class background. The connection to the college is informal but strong. Graduates of the college move back to the area for retirement; former professors and parents of current professors move to Winthrop House; residents take courses at the college; and professors give lectures at Winthrop House. Another strong link is to regional clergy, many of whom find their way to Winthrop House. The environment seems intellectual to me. Residents like a good academic lecture, and they form book clubs, poetry groups, and discussion circles. Being educated is part of the social glue and a rarefied trait of men and particularly women of this generation. So while the reputation is wrong based on cost alone, there is a distinct air of learnedness that may also affect who is attracted to or discouraged from joining Winthrop House. Finally, Winthrop House is also a destination for former and current employees. In 2012, nine residents had once worked at Winthrop House and six continued to work there.

Winthrop House residents are also from farther away than inhabitants of the other facilities in town. While most residents have personal connections to the Midwest, many have moved from remote places to retire at Winthrop House. Some have moved from the coasts to be closer to family members who are now living and working in the Midwest, others have researched excellent elder communities and decided on Winthrop House, and still others are connected to the local college, having worked at or attended it. Despite geographical diversity, Winthrop House is characterized by a white midwestern cultural milieu. So even if residents did not grow up in the Midwest, something about the social environment attracts them.

Racially and ethnically, the residents and workers of Winthrop House are less diverse than people in most parts of the United States and, in fact, are less diverse than the inhabitants of the surrounding region. Nearly all of the residents and over 90 percent of the workers are white and of European descent. Although a lower percentage of African American, Latino, Asian American, and American Indian elders than white elders live in CCRCs across the United States—as both a matter of choice and a matter of opportunity—the overwhelming number of white people at Winthrop House is very unusual. Across the United States, CCRC staffs are racially and ethnically diverse, often with workers of color filling the lesser-paid positions. Many facilities management, housecleaning, food service, and nursing aide staffs are made up of recent, nonwhite immigrants or refugees, as well as African American or Latina women and Latino men. While in most CCRCs many if not most of the workers are persons of color, this is not true at Winthrop House. Several residents pointed to the lack of racial diversity as one of the facility's weaknesses. When asked what would improve the place, they said that greater ethnic and racial diversity would benefit the community. Similarly, staff members occasionally check themselves in staff meetings to make sure that their assumptions about the kind of care residents want is not culturally specific to white midwestern or Christian values. However, these instances in which monoraciality becomes the subject of discussion are rare. While residents and staff alike proudly discuss the economic diversity, they are less likely to speak of the racial homogeneity that is also one of the defining characteristics of Winthrop House.

The facility offers a range of living options: independent living in built-to-specification duplex homes and apartments, assisted living, memory care for elders struggling with dementia or Alzheimer's disease, and a care center with 24/7 medical care. William King, the president, explains that Winthrop House is meant to provide flexible adjustments during times of change and transition.

> I guess the tagline is that we're a senior living and health care organization that intends to provide all the support one needs for living to the end of their life, and the goal is to live as long as one can independently, and when you reach the stage of not being able to, you have services available to you, whether they're rehab or long term.

Winthrop House advertises itself as a place where residents can live amid changing needs with readily available help at any level should their needs change over time. Even though residents hope not to need all the services, they report that the staged care is a major motivation for moving to Winthrop House.

The Winthrop House campus is large, covering ten square

blocks. Many residents said they moved to Winthrop House to get away from the chores of maintaining a private residence. Freedom from having to do shoveling, mowing, and other maintenance relieves a lot of concern and, as many residents report, affords them extra time to be busy in more meaningful and rewarding pursuits. One resident says that "most of the responsibility of maintaining a home is done for you, and you are free to enjoy the company of others." Another resident says she likes the "support when we need it, being left alone when we don't." She likens the facilities management staff to a son-in-law who comes anytime to help. Another resident says she is living a happy life and feels "protected, even coddled."

The staging of the spaces, opportunity to design one's own home or apartment, and beauty of the gardens are all described as primary attractions for potential residents. Residents can customize their apartments and houses to include open floor plans, stained-glass windows, patios, decks, and custom tubs. One resident describes the best part of living there as having the opportunity to "design our dream house!" Residents sit down with the home designer to decide on every detail. As I was passing out surveys, many residents invited me and my son in to see how they had arranged their space. Clearly, these personalized environments are a contrast to the institutional space many people imagine when they think of nursing homes. The opportunity to design one's own space also attracts a certain audience of people who may be used to a reasonably high degree of control over their living conditions. The approach communicates respect for individuality.

Similarly, the food service is set up to provide residents with flexible options. The quality, consistency, and convenience of the dining services are also noted as key aspects of Winthrop House's reputation and appeal. Residents appreciate that they do not have to buy a meal plan and instead can attend meals whenever it suits them. The dining service also willingly brings meals into the residences and even caters events for the residents to gather together or to host friends, family, or organizations to which they belong.

A tour through the Winthrop House campus begins at the striking gardens that are meticulously maintained by the facilities management staff and continues into common spaces, including clean and well-kept lounges, libraries, and entryways decorated in a rather unassuming fashion. Over the last twenty years, Winthrop House has worked to remove any semblance of design that reminds residents of hospitals or other institutional living quarters. Even in the care center—the most medicalized of all the living spaces—residents are encouraged to hang photos and bring their own TVs, radios, and easy chairs to make the space their own. Throughout the various levels of care, the walls have been papered, hardwood floors have been installed, and, when necessary, medical equipment has been tucked away to create a homey rather than a sterile medical environment. These design features have become the norm as elder care facilities seek to surprise potential residents with a homelike setting.

However, lacking major funding for a full teardown and replacement of some spaces, Winthrop House shows its age in the arrangement of space. Many workers long for a day when they can "start over" by building a facility that has even more generous spaces, wider hallways, and a circular arrangement of rooms (referred to in the industry as neighborhood style). With money to remodel, staff members imagine shared living rooms and kitchens for residents to cook in together rather than the long halls that currently house the most needy residents in the care center.

Despite the limitations set by building structures, Winthrop House staff work creatively to fulfill residents' desires. For example, in recent years, many of the residents moving in have asked for two apartments to be combined to allow for the more generous personal space to which they were accustomed in their original homes and condominiums. In the care center, where residents have twenty-four-hour nursing care, younger residents often request single rooms, so as current residents pass away or move out, the rooms are remodeled into singles to fulfill future demand. The administration has agreed to create these spaces even though such changes reduce the total number of spaces available. In staff meetings, workers are very aware of the changing interests and expectations of the next generation of people who will live at Winthrop House—the baby boomers. Within the limits of the budget, the administration works to offer flexible amenities, larger spaces, and greater opportunity for resident involvement as ways of satisfying current and prospective residents.

This Is Not Your Grandmother's Nursing Home

Ethnographic research often brings surprises. When one is getting to know a place, expectations can be upended. In the case of Winthrop House, I encountered three surprises. First, when I started observing and volunteering at Winthrop House, I was prepared to see daily life that looked a little like that of fish in a fish tank: slow on the surface with complexity that it takes a trained eye to recognize. I was quickly corrected in my expectation. Residents of Winthrop House are noticeably busy, exercising, leading organizations, planning events, and spending time together. Second, residents described their move to Winthrop House as an act of self-determination or an act of will. I was not prepared for this assertion because in many discussions about elder care facilities the move to one is described as a defeat. And finally, residents were not simply content; some were actively happy with their new home and the lifestyle it allows. I use these ethnographic surprises to provide snapshots of life at Winthrop House. I argue that residents' happiness stems from a feeling of being recognized and accompanied.

Residents do not sit around at home as I imagined they might. Instead, they are out in the world, so much so that it was difficult to track them down. To find out how they spent their busy days, I asked residents to describe an average day. Residents say that their lives are pleasantly busy. They recount opportunities to learn by taking courses at the local college, attending lecture series in town or at Winthrop House, and participating in one of the peer educational groups, including book clubs, a poetry club, and the campus newspaper. Residents also stay physically fit; many use the exercise room at Winthrop House, take the van for morning swimming at the local college, or walk the five blocks into the downtown area to run errands or visit friends.

Residents' descriptions of their lives contradict assumptions that elderly lives are passive. Residents talk about leadership positions they hold, political work they do, and their activism on the Winthrop House campus to get what they need for themselves and their neighbors. The boundaries that divide Winthrop House from the town are porous. In town, residents are involved in politics, faith organizations, volunteering, and civic organizations. Finally, residents keep busy with volunteer work, such as hosting international students, being volunteer grandparents, visiting elders in hospice care, transporting other residents who no longer drive, organizing events on the Winthrop House campus, or running fund drives at their church. Many residents keep in contact with family via Skype, e-mail, and phone, and a fair number maintain active home offices where they work daily.

These reports of what life is like run entirely counter to the very grim descriptions of nursing homes. While Winthrop House is not a nursing home per se, it houses the care center, which serves a nursing home function by providing round-the-clock care. And although residents certainly do not eagerly await a time when they will need the services of the care center, they say the availability of that kind of care is part of what motivated their move and what gives them peace of mind. In fact, they say that the care center was one of the criteria for their choice to move to Winthrop House.

The second surprise of my research was the degree of agency residents had exerted in their choice to move to Winthrop House. Their move was marked not by passivity or submission but by intentional planning that took their final years or decades out of the hands of others and into their own control. Settled now into their new lives, having done the difficult work of downsizing their homes and leaving neighborhoods behind, residents are happy where they live. Residents do not describe their move to Winthrop House as a compromise; instead, they view it as a way of exerting control, even agency, prior to what they imagine as future infirmities or limitations. Resident Wayne Milton explains that his children live too far away to be of assistance "day to day" as he and his wife get older, so "we wanted to relieve our children of the necessity of planning our future." Another resident, Mary Beth Kleinschmidt, says that when she got cancer, "I felt we should move while I was around to assist with leaving the big house—just in case I didn't live long. I am here and well twenty years later."

The duration of stay at Winthrop House speaks to the tendency among residents to make the move long before they find themselves in an active health crisis. While the average length of stay in a nursing home in the United States is eight hundred days, many residents of Winthrop House have lived there for ten, fifteen, even twenty years. Their much longer time at the facility gives them time to fully enjoy the services, connect with staff and new neighbors, and make new friends long before infirmity limits their socializing capacities.

Moving to Winthrop House is a way to arrange for the future, no matter what it might bring. A resident named Sally Jones summarizes how residents are alert to the challenges of elongated living and prolonged dying and how they choose proactively to embrace the move to Winthrop House as a way of resolving uncertainty and protecting loved ones.

> My husband of forty-eight years passed away in 2009. As time passed, I decided to move out of my home for the following reasons: I'm seventy years old and not knowing what the future holds for me, physically or mentally. Then if any physical problems should come up, my children won't have to get all concerned about putting me somewhere and trying to sell the house, et cetera. By my move here, I can go from beginning to end, and they won't have to worry about me, just love me.

By moving to Winthrop House on their own terms, residents get to make choices about their living environment prior to needing higher levels of care. Several residents moved to Winthrop House because a decline in their own or their spouse's health alerted them to the need for more help. Others made the move while feeling entirely well. Resident Bill Bumore explained that he moved as the result of "no special event—just awareness that I was aging and needed to take responsibility for myself." Similarly, Mick Rutley said that his move was inspired by "my acknowledgment of my aging process and my vulnerability." They feel that they have protected their children and other loved ones by not becoming dependent. Several residents described their move as having given a gift to their children by taking control of the later years of their lives.

This assertion of agency extends to how the residential community runs itself. Residents of Winthrop House are organized, politicized, and self-governing. They design programming; they run a governing organization, a charitable fund, a gift shop, and a volunteer network all within the ten-block campus. Within Winthrop House, residents exert more direct control over their living environment than in most elder care facilities: residents run their own association, which holds monthly meetings, operates separately from management, and makes and informs policy, as well as an advocacy committee, which provides companionship and keeps an eye out for the needs of less able residents. These advocates, who are residents themselves, volunteer to welcome new residents and accompany other residents through illness, periods of loss or grief, and moves to new spaces. The advocates meet to discuss their caseload and suggest new residents who might benefit from an advocate. Recently, the whole campus was alerted to a need when a single resident in independent living was stranded in his apartment for four days after a fall. Residents were understandably concerned about such an event recurring. They immediately organized a campus-wide buddy system for all single residents. Individually and collectively, residents are self-determining.

The third surprise for me was just how happy residents are with their surroundings. In direct contrast to harboring cultural fears that compare elder care facilities to asylums and prisons, residents of Winthrop House liken their daily close contact with similar-aged people to that experienced in college dorms. And, in fact, there is much about daily life that supports this comparison. The residents work to build connections with one another: they knock on one another's door in the morning, play games or work out in the afternoon, go for walks, attend talks, discuss books, and pick one another up to attend meals or programming together. Their days are punctuated by time spent deliberately in common. They plan to join one another for meals, stop to visit in one another's living space, pick one another up for activities, and celebrate birthdays and other milestones. They mark important moments in one another's lives in words and stories as well—gossiping, catching one another up on news, passing the word if someone is sick or ailing, and sharing good news and bad.

If Winthrop House is likened to a college campus, then it is a campus with sustained interactions between staff and residents. Administrator Ron Peattie says that one of the benefits for residents of the CCRC structure is that they are well known to the people who take care of them.

> How many of our management staff have been here over ten years? There is that sense of continuity that residents need. There is an advantage to coming to a retirement community where we know you as a person first, before you get known as a diagnosis. When you have a shared history, you tend to relate to people differently than people you've never met before.

Residents like that they know the staff by name and that when they need something, they are dealing with people they have known for a long while. The sense of mutual recognition is supported by the location in a small town—where residents and workers are known to one another in ways that extend beyond their roles in the CCRC. The community of Winthrop House is also made possible by the presence of both long-term residents and long-term staff. As Ron Peattie points out, staff members who have long tenure in their positions and approach their work as a vocation earn the trust of residents. In the local economy, a position at Winthrop House is a quality job that workers are hesitant to leave. For example, dining services director Clark Daily reports that many workers in dining service have been in their jobs since the

1980s, having put in as many as thirty years of service. Winthrop House has very low turnover, even among entry-level positions such as nurse's aide jobs. While the average turnover in the industry is 100 percent, at Winthrop House the turnover is less than 40 percent. Several nurse's aides have worked at Winthrop House for more than a decade. Many employees plan to never leave by becoming residents themselves. At the time of this writing, fifteen residents were former or current employees of Winthrop House.

The social spaces between residents and staff are short: there is little pretense, and participants recognize and assist one another with life's ups and downs. Residents also routinely extend interest in, curiosity about, and attention to staff and their families. Residents and staff are informal in their interactions with one another. They refer to one another by name, they inquire about one another's families, staff members bring in children to visit the residents, and residents introduce family members to staff members. Name tags emphasize the first names of staff members, and all conversations are conducted on a first-name basis, with the exception of the rare resident who prefers to be addressed more formally. Cards and gifts are exchanged, homemade treats are shared, compliments are paid, and concern is conveyed. Residents' and staff members' sense of commonality is also likely facilitated by the unusual monoraciality that characterizes the place: the sameness of residents and staff in terms of race and birthplace may be part of the foundation for familiarity. Although being white is not a quality that residents or staff point to as part of the social glue at Winthrop House, it is a defining feature. As such, it must appeal to or at least be tolerable to residents who have multiple choices about where to live. When the facility becomes more diverse, as some members hope it will, it should become clear how large a role monoraciality plays in sustaining the easy mutual recognition that exists.

On the surface, workers at Winthrop House help residents with nursing needs connected to illness and activities of daily living (ADLs), and they provide home maintenance, food service, social activities, and entertainment. Those functional matters sustain bodies and minds, but on a philosophical and even practical level what workers spend much of their time doing is helping residents through life's final transitions. This kind of assistance is particularly important because workers' expertise and attention are applied to a time of life that is undervalued and undersupported in many social environments in the United States. If there is one practice that epitomizes what workers labor to do, it is the work of easing transition.

Help in Times of Transition

As residents move to Winthrop House, social worker Rita Sanford and the direct care providers work to get to know the resident and his or her preferences, daily needs, and likes.

> [We need] to establish that trust and have them figure out who I am and what we're all about and hav[e] them begin to trust their caregivers. So, again, my background doing that and knowing that is so essential. For me, the first few days, I want to know "How are you sleeping? Is the bed okay? Do you like to take an evening bath? Do you like to have butter-brickle ice cream at seven o'clock before you go to bed?" So we begin the communication. . . . Once I get to know all of that, then you pass that down [to other staff members] so that it can be delivered.

Once day-to-day care is established, Phyllis Star, the chaplain, reaches out to the resident and family members to begin conversations about the resident's spiritual and practical desires and to help them think about transitions before they occur.

> So, [in] one of my conversations sometimes, I *will* ask, "What is the meaning of your life? What are the goals for the *rest* of your life?" Some people, sometimes they need to just chat and laugh, and they want to check out what's going on in the world . . . linking them with people and resources, connecting them with staff sometimes.

While Chaplain Star encourages family members and residents to engage in planning relating to goals and faith, nurse Nikki Johnson describes it as her job to help family members recognize physical changes early on and initiate discussion of such changes so that she can put measures in place to ease those transitions. She explains that she will say, "We're seeing a decline. I want to prepare you for this. Let's talk about what you see for the future for Mom or Dad. What would you like to be, in terms of where we're at, if we're going to move them, you know?" Staff use their knowledge of residents combined with their accrued knowledge from training and work experience to help residents and their family members anticipate upcoming needs.

Once residents have lived at Winthrop House for a period of time, they begin to develop habits and routines in their new space. The next level of care builds on those routines by helping to sustain satisfying routines, offer new opportunities, and watch for changes. Clark Daily, who runs food services, gives an example of how his department is well positioned to notice changes in residents. Since mealtime offers daily points of contact between dining services and residents, he and his staff are attentive to changes in residents' movements, appetite, and outlook. He explains how he and his staff might start a conversation with a resident or tip off the medical staff so that adjustments can be made. As Clark explains, residents sometimes try to mask changes in their health because they do not want to have to move, especially to the care center, which is viewed as a place to be avoided because it is often perceived as the last stop before death.

> A lot of [residents] know that something's going on with them. They know there's a change, but [they cover it up] because a lot of them have a huge fear of the care center, you know. They don't want to end up across the street. Well, just because you're sick or something along those lines doesn't mean you're going to end up there. But especially if there's something you can do to prevent that, you know, in your apartment.

When Daily notices such a change, he brings his observations to the interdisciplinary staff meeting. The staff can then work together to provide additional assistance when needed without forcing the resident to move or lose a sense of self-worth or self-control. At these meetings, workers get together to think creatively about individual residents' needs over time. One story that illustrates this work is that of Gerald Fullbright.

Gerald Fullbright started out at Winthrop House eight years ago in an independent living apartment. When he became more frail and needed help with some ADLs, he and his family decided he should transfer to the assisted living part of Winthrop House. This move turned out to be a happy one for Gerald. He enjoyed the planned activities, became friendly with two of the other men on his floor, and liked having his meals provided. If anything, his health seemed to improve initially.

After three years in the assisted living environment, Gerald was taken to the emergency room to get his vomiting and blood pressure under control. His hospital stay was expected to be short. While he was still in the hospital, Gerald's case became the topic of discussion at an interdisciplinary staff meeting. These meetings take place every three weeks and include representatives from each department and across a range of training and background. In attendance are members of the top administration, the director of nursing, the head of nursing in each building, the social worker, the home health director, the chaplains, the billing staff, and the heads of the facilities management and dining service departments. The subject matter of these meeting—which run between one and three hours—is the residents. The sole document used is a list of residents who are undergoing transition, and their care then becomes the topic of conversation. Some residents are discussed for half an hour and others for a couple of minutes. On the day that staff members brought up Gerald's case at such a meeting, they did so because they felt that when he came back from the hospital, they would need to think about helping Gerald make the next move to the care center. William King, the president of Winthrop House, said that one of the employees who was leaving—Candi Richard— had a connection with the family, who had known her when she was young. King noted that they would have to replace Candi as the key contact person with the family.

As the group discussed Gerald's recent past and the next few months, many of the people around the table used terms such as *plateaus* and *precipitous decline*. The progress that Gerald made in his early years in assisted living had ended, and he was growing sicker, more tired, and less interested in daily activities. The group discussed the need to be "proactive" with family and friends in order to let them know what they had observed and to prepare them for the fact that Gerald might not simply return to his apartment. As they had prior to his last move into assisted living, staff members observed that Gerald was down; he seemed more pensive than usual. The one thing that he truly enjoyed was visits from volunteers with animals and especially the cat that lived in the memory wing. Staff explored ways to connect Gerald with the cat more often when he returned from the hospital. They believed that integrating something pleasurable like time with the cat might make the next move more appealing for Gerald as well. Gerald's story reveals the sustained attention to individuals, the incorporation of various forms of expertise in the care of residents, and the intentional use of institutional memory that having long-term staff members allows. The people around the table knew Gerald and remembered him, they recognized his preferences, and they planned ahead with and for him, even as he recovered in a hospital room off campus.

The long tenure of staff members makes recognition at Winthrop House a reality. Such recognition is incredibly important later in life because elders like Gerald are increasingly reliant on the good intentions of caregivers and their knowledge of the elders as individuals. At Winthrop House, an organizational structure—the interdisciplinary staff meeting—deliberately encircles residents who are undergoing changes with the attention, observations, and skills of workers from a range of specialties. Interactions over a period of years lay the groundwork for individualized care plans that recognize residents' unique preferences, capacities, and tendencies, and this recognition can be crucial. Imagine a person who recently lost her life partner—who could finish her sentence and anticipate her needs. Imagine the comfort of being offered a favorite meal, of having the cat brought in to cheer you, or of daily visits from a friendly face as you settle into a new home. Staff members cannot replace loved ones who are lost, the less "condensed" environments of previous homes, or the more robust abilities of younger bodies and minds, but they can offer recognition and familiarity through the twists and turns of aging.

When one ill resident returned from a hospital stay, dining services director Clark Daily did not even have to ask what the resident wanted for her welcome-home meal. He knew that her favorite food was hash browns and sausage patties. Clearly, such acts of recognition do not mitigate physical pain if it is present, but what familiarity *does* mitigate is the potential anonymity and loneliness that being "institutionalized" might entail in an environment where residents are not recognized as unique individuals. This ability to anticipate is like the work that family members do for loved ones; the special touches ease the difficult days by committing to memory what one craves or enjoys.

Given the cultural similarities of the residents, the question remains if such recognition could be as easily extended in a more diverse environment. What if a resident's favorite food was arroz con pollo or grits and greens? Can dining services provide comforting foods derived from tastes and experiences that are not white, midwestern, or Christian? While the scope of recognition has yet to be fully explored, in the meantime, being able to provide recognition is a source of pride for workers and benefits residents during the final chapters of their lives.

Company in Death's Long Shadow

Underlying the buzz of activity at Winthrop House is a series of challenges that workers and residents cooperate to address. There are the usual challenges of living in close proximity: old loves and hatreds, acts of exclusion or intolerance, sharing of common space and resources. The age specificity of Winthrop House's inhabitants also presents challenges concerning autonomy, security, individuality, collectivity, and identity. This community is a fragile accomplishment. Sustaining the sense of community means finding ways to feel connected amid loss and to keep one another company in the long shadow of death's approach.

Resident Martha Beckman says, "So far as I can tell, Winthrop House has created and sustained in its residents a strong sense of mutual purpose, interest, and joy in living here. That's not to say, of course, that we don't also share our gripes and worries." One of the primary worries of residents is the challenge of death's presence. Agnes and Harley French both feel that the age segregation of their community presents unique challenges. When I asked them what the most challenging aspect of living at Winthrop House was, Agnes replied, "good friends dying," and Harley said, "coping with the aging process and doing it with as much grace and dignity as you see in others." Like the Frenches, many residents speak to the challenges of living in an age-specific community that makes death a more common experience. Resident Harlo Hayward summarizes this challenge.

> Without a doubt, being a member of the Winthrop House community makes you continually aware of mortality. Over forty residents died last year, and I think that's a regular number. Two people I played bridge with regularly died in the last six months. Three or four people I've gotten to know at lunch have had to move to assisted living or the care center, and there are at least four people I know who are experiencing dementia problems. It's part of life here.

As Harlo explains, death is unavoidable at Winthrop House in ways that are less true beyond those ten square blocks. Many of the buffers in place that protect people from the inevitability of death and old age are stripped away in the CCRC setting.

The pressures and worries that accompany being in a community with higher levels of infirmity, decline due to aging, and death than in the general population are not purely bad. Residents explain that they learn from observing how their friends and neighbors navigate the changes that occur in old age. Resident Elizabeth Simmons explains that she struggles with "being confronted with so many folks with diminishing capabilities." Elizabeth's notion of "being confronted" clearly explains the dilemma: with closeness comes intimate knowledge of others' changes, both for better and for worse. The benefit is that frank discussion of aging and death is routine practice at Winthrop House, while the downside is that elders are confronted with a possible vision of their own future. This confrontation may motivate positive choices, but it can also haunt their imaginations to have close contact with other people who are dying.

Residents describe their private struggles with the downside of the longevity dividend: the possibility that longer lives and slower deaths will entail a loss of control, uncontrolled dependency, and, in short, misery. They worry about living "too long" under conditions not of their choosing and about the circumstances of their own future death. Resident Mary Beth Kleinschmidt explains that she worries she will not react to her own aging as she needs to or she will lose the support she relies on: "I worry I won't want to give up the things I expect other residents to give up as they age. I'll hang on to my car too long; I won't want to give up living in an independent living home and go to a small apartment: I will lose Thomas, or he won't be able to take care of me." When I asked a resident named Phil Dwyer how life at Winthrop House measured up to his expectations, he said his expectations had been exceeded. However, he added, "The bumps in the road of aging were not expected and much harder to accept than I had imagined." Phil's observation represents a sentiment shared by many residents: life at Winthrop House is good; for some, it's as good as it gets, but that does not alter some of the fears of the conditions of later life. The place they live provides them with resiliency and security, yet the conditions of old age and death can still be a source of fear and dread. As resident Shirley Cousins explains, "I don't have many concerns except for the one major one that most of us here at Winthrop House have—that is, how much longer will relatively good health continue?" Their home comforts them; how we die now troubles them.

Residents worry about becoming a burden to their children or spouses, about outliving their financial reserves, and about being in pain. Most of all, residents worry about living beyond what they consider quality of life. As resident Mary Westchester says, "At age ninety-five (ninety-six soon!), I don't have much of a 'future,' but I would rather 'go' than sit around in a wheelchair and my brain not working." Other residents say they do not want to "linger long" when the time comes to die and they hope to "avoid a long, drawn-out dying process." Sandy Madrid explains the fears she and her husband have and the efforts they are making to stave off their biggest concerns.

> We worry about the possibility of losing our minds before we die, and using up much of the money we have set aside to leave to our two children—neither of whom have any pension—for additional help at the care center. We are now in the process of planning our funerals by outlining our life histories and choosing material to include in the services. With one child in Asia and the other [on the coast], and no other close relatives, we have to think about these things.

Resident Martha Montgomery says she hopes that "my money does not run out and that I have a short, fast, painless death." Another resident, Barb Resin, reflects humorously on the almost universal desire to die in one's sleep. "My 'choice' is to slip away peacefully in my bed some night—HAH—likely thought!" For these elders, worse things can happen than death itself. While death is inevitable and planned on, residents work to put in place protections against the other kinds of losses they might suffer.

Being involved in an aged community seems to have empowered residents to be particularly clear about what they do and do not want when their own death comes. Having lived long enough to witness many deaths, they are sure about what they are prepared to face and what they would count as a travesty. While Mary Beth Kleinschmidt worries she will lose her husband, Thomas, or make bad choices as her health declines, Thomas fears that he will somehow get dragged into what he sees as the fruitless pursuit of a longer life using extreme medical interventions at the end of life. He explains, "I deplore how some cling to 'do everything possible.' In my opinion, this leads to diminished quality of life and much expense that I feel is unjustified and borderline unethical." Resident Sara Titan summarizes what she has learned and subsequently decided from her time at Winthrop House.

> My main concerns are that the ending of my life . . . not involve a prolonged period of helplessness, nor create an undue burden or anxiety for my children. I think that living at Winthrop House helps me prepare for the stages to come in my aging. I am inspired by the lives of my fellow residents, particularly the wisdom and courage which they exhibit in so many different ways.

Residents hope for the opportunity to age gracefully and to die peacefully. In their pursuit of these goals, their fates intersect in important ways with the intentions and actions of Winthrop House staff.

Protection without Paternalism

All the changes at the end of life shift the locus of control between the residents and the people who care for them: both family members and staff members. At times, staff need to develop ways of protecting residents from themselves, from complications of their illnesses, and sometimes even from family members. The staff work together to try to offer protective care that is not paternalistic. The more help a resident needs, the more risk there is that staff will intentionally or unintentionally tread on a resident's autonomy. As he explains what Winthrop House can offer residents, administrator Ron Peattie says, "We've had a chance to interact in each other's lives," and he talks about avoiding paternalism, describing it as the tension between what he calls security and interference.

> This is a way of life more than it is a place to live. Residents feel secure, and we as staff try to maintain that separation between security and interference. We're providing tangible means of safety, security, nutrition, health care to the people in this [community]. There is a sense of cooperation, a sense of sharing—the residents are very generous in their time, in their finances. It's like a town unto itself—it's a self-contained community. We're neighbors. We're steady family. It's a genuine bond of affection and connectedness.

The goal, as Peattie explains it, is to provide a self-contained community without creating an environment that is overdetermined or sealed off from possibility. Staff members do not want security to come at the cost of choice or pleasure. Behind the scenes of everyday life, staff members deliberate with one another about how to calibrate the balance between safety and freedom. Two examples of this delicate balance came up during interdisciplinary staffing meetings. They involved one resident's nightly walks and another's love of gardening.

In the first instance, the desire to have locked doors after 8:00 P.M. for residents' sense of security was weighed against the interest of Dolores McDaniel, who took walks at night and sometimes, because of dementia, forgot the alternative routes back into the building when she did not bring her key. At Winthrop House, the apartment buildings are locked at night so that only people with keys can enter after that time. One spring morning, the interdisciplinary staffing meeting took up the question of Dolores's evening walks. In doing so, they weighed the collective interest in security against the individual security of the resident who sometimes forgot how to access an unlocked path of reentry. Staff had twice witnessed Dolores's need for assistance in reentering the building safely. This was not an unacceptable situation in the springtime, but they worried it could become more dangerous in the coming months as the weather became colder. When a chaplain ran into her on the street, Dolores did not have the key to her apartment. Asked how she would get back inside, Dolores knew she could reenter through the unlocked care center but was less clear about the directions to that facility. The chaplain helped her but worried about a repeat of the situation in inclement weather. During the day, Dolores was fit, physically able, and perfectly capable of navigating her way through Winthrop House with ease. However, like other people with minor dementia, Dolores occasionally thought less clearly at night, so what she might know easily at noon was less obvious to her at 8:00 P.M., when she liked to go for her walk. Among their solutions, staff considered unlocking the door closest to her residence, asking Dolores to walk earlier in the evening, and locking the doors later in the evening. The ultimate solution was to involve a neighbor to walk with her or keep an eye out to make sure she had an easy way back into the building, particularly during inclement weather. Dolores's situation is an example of a straightforward challenge of collective living. If Dolores lived with family members, they too would have had to think about how to honor her desire to walk. In this case, her desire had to be weighed against the preferences of the other fifteen people who lived in her building. The strong connections between staff and residents made it possible to limit the intrusion into her freedom by asking a neighbor to subtly help to keep her safe.

The second instance was much more complicated to resolve. It involved a resident named Henry Farrell who loved to garden. He kept busy carrying dirt and water in buckets to prepare his summer garden. Henry had gardened his whole life and was very adept at all aspects of preparing the earth, monitoring the plants, and harvesting flowers and food. He came to the attention of the staff meeting because he had fallen on uneven ground while gardening, and so one of the nurses wondered if the facilities management staff could assist Henry with some of the more physical demands of his work. Facilities staff talked with Henry to assess his willingness to share the labor, but he was adamantly opposed to assistance in creating the garden—it was the activity that brought him the most pleasure. Chaplain Phyllis Star reported that she had found him out in the garden in a huge wind and had commented to Henry that the wind might blow him away. Henry replied, "I've been in the wind my whole life." Social worker Rita Sanford said that life always involves risk, and Michael Wood, head of the facilities staff, concluded the discussion by saying, "Henry has been in the dirt his whole life, people." The discussion of safety quickly digressed into a more philosophical consideration of roots, pursuits, and passions. Staff members demonstrated a deep respect for the resident and his pursuits, and they saw themselves in him.

Their shared interest was in facilitating Henry's gardening; the only question was how best to do so. They wanted to avoid allowing the institution to override Henry's right to pursue activities that gave him pleasure. Implicitly, the discussion was also about risk and when there is a risk worth taking.

Deliberation about Henry's gardening concluded after Wood said, "If you take that away from him, he will die. He was born with the wind in his hair, and he needs to have his hands in the earth. We can't take that work away from him." The tension here between security and autonomy and the risk of being paternalistic were much more intense than in the case of Dolores. Do you allow residents to continue to complete tasks that have an element of danger for aging bodies but that bring them pleasure? When do you decide that safety is more important than joy and a sense of accomplishment? After much discussion, a general consensus in support of Wood's point—that gardening was an essential activity for this resident—developed. It was a risk that Henry himself recognized and embraced. They resolved to leave Henry alone to do the things that brought him pleasure despite the risks.

At Winthrop House the interdisciplinary staff meeting provides a context for staff members to deliberate about difficult choices. Such choices are potential crossroads—moments when the balance of power between residents and staff is negotiated. The issues they debate mark the dilemmas posed by elongated lives—dilemmas many of us will face when we age, whether we live in an aged community or not: moments of decision about whether we can keep doing the activities that have defined us and helped shape our lives, whether it is our nightly walk at 8:00 P.M. or hauling dirt and water. If we age at home, then we deliberate these choices alone, with spouses, or with children. In the CCRC setting, these choices become the subject of both personal and institutional decision making within the limits of regulatory compliance. Sometimes staff can be a force of constraint and con-servatism, encouraging residents to rethink their routines, while at other times staff can be a source of experience and creativity, help-ing residents maintain their daily practices under slightly altered conditions.

The decisions made by the interdisciplinary staffing commit-tee are directions to pursue, not end, goals. Once the staff mem-bers have deliberated, a "point person" is identified who moves forward with the plan to talk with the residents, present options, or seek assistance from additional sources, such as Dolores's neigh-bor. Staff members debate these dilemmas with what appears to be a genuine interest in the most expansive notion of resident auton-omy. For example, in a facility governed by regulatory bodies, the fact that the interdisciplinary staff meeting had openly discussed the risks that Henry took to maintain his gardening paradoxically put the facility at risk: if he fell during an activity they had previ-ously identified as risky, Winthrop House could be subject to fines, penalties, and additional inspections. Staff members were aware of this institutional risk but were unwilling to confine Henry for rea-sons of regulatory compliance. In the end, Ron Peattie concluded the discussion by saying, "I can live with a stain on our inspection if it means Henry gets to keep gardening for another couple of seasons." The respect afforded the residents in these discussions is noteworthy—it lacks the paternalism that many associate with elder care facilities. Most of all, the infantilization of old people so prevalent in parts of American culture seems to be absent here. The deliberations of this group reveal their commitments to living on the level with the residents. The respect that residents feel in face-to-face interactions with staff continues behind the scenes at staff meetings. This consistency of mission—sustaining an elderly community—grounds daily practice at Winthrop House. In addi-tion to engendering many positive outcomes, residents' relationship to staff and to Winthrop House itself can create new tensions regarding intimacy, family, and authority.

Stories Never Told

In addition to raising questions about security and autonomy, old age raises questions about authority and who we can trust to have power over us. Who will take care of us? Who will make decisions for us when we can no longer decide for ourselves? Who can be trusted to usher us toward death? These concerns are actively taken up in the Winthrop House context. While residents may feel loyal to and supported by staff, residents' family members may struggle to trust paid workers to care for their loved ones. Fears of aging, mistrust of market-based relationships, and beliefs about elder care facilities may all inform family members' hesitancy to partner with staff members in the care of the residents.

Even when it is based on the choice of the resident, the move into Winthrop House represents a double-edged opportunity for new connections at the possible expense of old connections. Specifically, the authority of family members based on a long and intimate history with the resident is now joined and maybe challenged by the professional authority and expertise of staff members who also come to know the resident well. Having witnessed and accompanied others through these important transitions, staff members are attuned to some of the changes that can be anticipated, and if their expertise is acknowledged, they can help residents or their family members adjust to the transitions under way. New connections between staff and residents can be a source of comfort, but they can also raise tensions with family members, particularly with regard to decision making, power, and trust.

One of the underlying beliefs that support the fear of nursing homes is that as an elder becomes increasingly dependent and increasingly unable to make decisions, support should be found in only family networks or very old friendships. The fears that so often encompass elder care facilities have their counterparts in the valuation of familial networks as the *preferable* locations for elder care. Accompanying this is an often unarticulated belief that kinship will protect against abuse and neglect. In this view, reliance on paid care providers is profane. The idea is that the familial tie, particularly a blood relation, provides the best way to know and fulfill elders' wishes at the end of life. Moving into an elder care facility represents a (sometimes unrecognized) choice to share that locus of control, that site of expertise, and, often, that burden.

For residents and their family members, entry into Winthrop House is the first of many step-by-step adjustments as the family modifies the responsibility for care: they share the weight of caregiving, and over time, they often share intimate knowledge of the care recipient. Staff members come to know the residents well and differently from the way family members do. Combined with staff members' experience and training, this familiarity becomes a basis for recommendations and sometimes decisions about the best way to assist residents with changes in their health and needs. But family members often distrust the authority of paid caregivers, and, reciprocally, staff members sometimes come to question the intentions of certain family members. The shared condition of caregiving can create sites of conflict related to authority.

Although it is practically a sacrilege to say in our culture, my observations at Winthrop House have led me to believe that living in a community of similarly aged neighbors that is staffed by experts on aging and dying offers some *advantages* over care at home by family members. In order to make a case for the advantages of such an arrangement, I need to tell the sort of stories that staff members are reluctant to share—stories about the tensions between family care and institutional care.

Most of us are death novices. When we are trying to help a loved one navigate reduced mobility, losses in function, chronic pain, restlessness, frustration, and prolonged defeat to multiple diseases, we are out of our league. Sometimes when family members are in these unknown waters, we make decisions that are less than apt. Even worse, sometimes families make mistakes or abuse or neglect their loved ones. The reasons for those circumstances are many and may be related to family strain, old disagreements, a lack of material resources, and genuine ignorance. My point here is not to indict families; it is, rather, to shift the story a bit from what elder care facilities do wrong to what they do right and, more specifically, to the mishaps and missteps that can be identified and maybe even avoided when the "village" that cares for an elder at the end of life includes both loving novices and trained experts.

Unlike the stories told directly to me in interviews, these stories were either observed or overheard; because they are taboo, they were not related explicity. Particularly at Winthrop House, where residents and staff cooperate to emphasize the positive, these stories reveal ruptures. I also opt not to present these tales in interviews because I would consider it offensive to show staff justifying work that they consider meaningful by pointing to the errors and transgressions of families. Unlike horror stories of elder abuse or neglect in institutional care, rarely do these stories of how elder care facilities insert themselves meaningfully into dying processes move beyond the walls of the facility.

In the first case, members of one wealthy family refused to pay for increased care for their elderly mother who was confined to bed. At the interdisciplinary staff meeting, participants deliberated about how to convince the family that more staff coverage was needed to maintain her quality of life: she was unable to seek help if something was wrong because she could not use or reach a phone. She was often found left for hours in wet adult diapers with no one to change her, and she was locked in her home with no system for assistance. In short, she was not only bed bound; she was actually trapped in her bed because she lacked assistance. At first, staff worried that her family had failed to increase support because they had not come to terms with her decline, but as the months passed and the inaction continued, they became concerned that the family was willfully neglecting to improve staffing coverage in order to save money. The staff members quietly debated whether or not they had the power to take control of a resident in independent living. In other words, they wondered if they could exercise control over the resident that would *trump* the family's inaction.

In the second case, family members willfully overrode an order not to sustain the life of a resident. The resident persisted in a vegetative state for years against the wishes he had expressed in his advance directive. Meanwhile, the person with the medical power of attorney lived in his house and collected his pension. Staff members struggled for years to find an alternative legal approach to fulfill the resident's last known wishes.

In a third case, staff members expressed concern about a resident who could no longer care for her husband. They watched as her health declined precipitously and her husband refused to seek or pay for outside assistance. She was too frail to move him, and yet he required regular bodily cares. She broke bones, lost weight, and appeared increasingly despondent. Her daughters, who visited twice a month, were proud of the close bond their parents shared, while staff members fretted for weeks, then months, as they watched the wife decline rapidly under the strain of her caregiving burden.

In broad strokes, these are the heartbreaking choices that take place within the ten square blocks that make up Winthrop House.

Where is the proper line between paid and unpaid caregivers? What is interference, and what is assistance? What are the responsibilities of community members if some of those bonds are based in blood and some in paid caregiving?

Retelling these stories is meant to acknowledge just how messy the end of life can be in terms of trust, changes in function, and shared responsibility. I have watched with admiration as staff members have tried to manage these complexities. These stories also highlight just how difficult sustaining the dream of staying at home can be. Families struggle beneath the enormous pressures, complexity, and constant changes that accompany prolonged dying. Although most Americans hope to age and then die in their own homes, the conditions of longer lives sometimes make keeping up with the changes difficult, even with the assistance of paid care providers.

My point here is to try to capture some of the grace and insight that the workers at Winthrop House bring to the work that they do. Their care and perspective can never *replace* the care of family members, but more often than not, these offerings can be a meaningful supplement to the many transitions associated with old age in the contemporary era. That partnership between staff, residents, and their family members can provide a basis for a well-planned conclusion to one's life.

Learning from Life at Winthrop House

When it comes to this elder boom, I think of a childhood rallying cry, "Ready or not, here we come!" This demographic shift cannot be bargained with—it is coming. In fact, it is already under way. Our country is graying. Will we experience this graying reluctantly, or will we meet the challenges directly? If I were single-handedly in charge, I would build an army of well-trained, well-paid home health providers who take care of elders across a range of abilities. This army of well-rewarded workers would make sure that elders could age and die at home as they say they want to.

My research on aging has taught me that even if we had this army of workers, some elders would likely change their minds about being at home because some of the major diseases that kill us now ravage the body in ways that make institutional care a needed relief. For elders wrestling with such diseases, institutional care is nothing to rail against. In fact, as we become an aged society, it makes no sense to vilify an institution that specializes in caring for elders as they move into old age and active dying. Winthrop House is just one of the tens of thousands of elder care facilities in the United States. It is a distinctive place, shaped by its specific location and social context. It is a place where residents and workers have agreed to explore the new territory made possible by the longevity dividend willingly. Some even are living out their old age gleefully. In the search for organizations, institutions, guidance, and assistance in the coming decades, Winthrop House may be an unusually healthy environment. Certainly there are CCRCs and nursing homes where residents are not as satisfied, but there are other "Winthrop Houses"—pleasant places where residents and workers labor together to get the work of aging and dying done meaningfully.

Examining participants' stories can tell us some things that are generalizable about aging and community in early twenty-first-century American life, while other aspects of Winthrop House are distinct to the particular context in which participants play their parts. Local dynamics combine with dynamics specific to elder communities, including unpredictable changes in health and the regular attrition of community members due to death. The age-specific dynamics of elder living combine with the particulars of this place—specifically, the culture of optimism, the long tenure of staff, the dominance of white people in the space, and the integration of staff and family members into what participants call the "community" of Winthrop House—to shape day-to-day interactions.

At best, communities are places that anticipate and fulfill our needs and provide us with opportunities to pay into a communal pot of material and emotional resources. Members of communities find a space that feels more homey, more familiar, where members can feel a sense of ownership for the interactions and practices that make up that social space. Finally, communities remember their members: our presence in a communal space is not immediately erased; we leave a mark that is recalled after our departure. By necessity, many of the rituals that characterize everyday life at Winthrop House include this kind of mutual recollection: replaying memories of friends, family, and neighbors who have left the space through death and even preparing for the loss of those community members who are actively dying, whose time within the space is short. While certainly members of Winthrop House struggle to talk about death gracefully, the routine acknowledgment of mortality is a key characteristic, reflecting a more frank negotiation with death than in the larger culture that surrounds the space, but the constancy of death can take a toll.

This community is a fragile accomplishment—it takes sustained commitment and trust between all the groups that shape daily life there. Even small ruptures in that trust could alter the social environment. New demands made by the next generation of elders may create different strains, and as the United States becomes increasingly diverse in terms of race, ethnicity, and faith, and more bifurcated in terms of class, some of the tensions raised by those differences might introduce new strains. Residents and staff value what they have enough that concerns about dislodging the comfortable coexistence come up in many conversations.

In some ways, protecting what they see as a rare environment might be part of what feeds each group's affirmations about life at Winthrop House. Residents and staff rally around this place because they view it as special and worthy of defending. For residents, Winthrop House provides a final community in which they feel recognized and supported. For staff, Winthrop House presents work that is demanding, makes use of their skills, and provides them with an arena to make a difference in people's lives and to feel proud of their work. From their interactions with elder individuals who are navigating their mortality, staff members also learn many things about life. It is to these lessons we now turn.

4

Lessons from the End of Life

What Workers Learn from Helping Others Die

Helping other people die is physically, medically, emotionally, socially, and spiritually demanding. Those who do the work also describe it as rewarding. When I interviewed a family care provider named Janet Conroy, I ended our discussion by asking what advice she would give to someone who was just beginning to care for an elder person. Janet described her involvement with her mother's last years as a rite of passage—one that left her stronger, more assured, and grateful:

> It's such a big life experience. It really is. To have experienced it, it literally changed me, and I feel like I'm so much better for it. I honestly feel like I had a problem with what I called existential loneliness. [Prior to this] I was just one of those people who was always lonely. And honestly, after all this, it was as if it just dropped away—I have not had that feeling since. It feels like I never knew what I was standing on before, but after this experience I feel like I'm always

literally standing on a rock. I'm on such a firm foundation, it's just not shakable. It was really hard getting through it. . . . There were moments where I was encouraged by a couple of people—my husband was one of them—to take something to take the edge off of it. And I said, "If I take the edge off of it, I'm going to miss something. So, sorry, you have to deal with it." [*Giggles.*] Because, you know, the anxiety comes up, the worry comes up, but if I'm going to have an experience like this in my life and I don't learn about how to deal with anxiety and worry and putting things aside, where am I? I had trouble sleeping, but I was like, "Well, I'll learn how to sleep." And I did. It wasn't easy, but it was really worthwhile. And now, I don't worry to the point where I can't sleep, because everything seems so small in comparison to that. I'm like, eh, if I can [help my mom die], I can do this. There are moments where I occasionally feel a little bit guilty that I got so much out of it; I'm thinking, I hope my mother doesn't mind that I used her experience for me.

Janet Conroy expresses gratitude for having been there beside her mother, for having experienced the process fully, and, finally, for having had the privilege of helping her do the work of wrapping up her life. Janet describes herself as altered by the opportunity. The experience made Janet more self-assured and more certain of her priorities. Many people who accompany others toward death talk about the changes in themselves. They describe awful moments during the ravages of illness and impending death, but they also report gratitude for having been a witness, having accompanied the person they cared for into death. Janet takes this even further; she herself feels accompanied and less lonely as a result of her experience with her mother's death. What Janet describes is a kind of competence that she acquired from the work of caring for her mother, and she carries the confidence and calm that she developed during that process with her, even now, years after her mother's death. In this chapter, I explore the ways of knowing and doing developed by all the people who make a living by assisting others in the final days and months of their lives. Like Janet, they have developed concrete skills and consistent beliefs about their work—I call these discoveries arising from their work *lessons from the end of life*.

While previous chapters have focused on the day-to-day *living* in elder communities, I turn now to another aspect of elder care facilities: dying. Elder communities are not like hotels because for the most part residents do not check out. The average length of stay in an elder care community is 835 days (Centers for Disease Control and Prevention 2011). At the end of that time, the vast majority of elders die. As such, death is more common in elder communities than in age-diverse communities. For workers in elder care facilities, death is part of the continual context of their work. End-of-life workers are pioneers in the social environment that now accompanies end-of-life processes, yet they are rarely recognized for or consulted about what they know.

Every occupation produces a set of specialized knowledge. Occupational insiders know the aspects of their work that are taken for granted well enough that they begin to treat their expertise like common sense, making use of highly specialized facts as if they were self-evident (Smith 1988). Newcomers to occupational cultures are quick to identify and then attempt to acquire the specialized knowledge that insiders possess. Part of "learning the ropes" in a new profession entails coping strategies and techniques that contain the costs and improve the quality of work for the worker (Fillion, Fortier, and Goupil 2005; Irurita and Williams 2001). Waiters and waitresses share techniques for earning higher tips, while hospice and nursing home workers share techniques for working in the shadow of mortality. Like other forms of occupational know-how, death competence (Gamino and Ritter 2009: 31) captures a kind of certainty that is comforting, is professionally advantageous, and allows end-of-life workers to feel proud of their work. From high-status workers such as managers, doctors, and chaplains to low-status workers such as house cleaners, food servers, and nurse's aides, service providers acquire ways of thinking about and responding to the dying process that attempt to manage the shock of mortality (Walter 1994).

Living in a culture that supports incompetence rather than knowledge and awareness about death and dying, many Americans could benefit from access to the special lessons that death experts can teach us about how we die now. Many Americans face their own or their loved ones' death uninformed about the forces shaping the dying process in our current historical moment. Knowledge and experience with death are particularly valuable at a time when dying persons and their families have to answer difficult questions, such as: Should I try to keep Mom at home? Does my husband want to be resuscitated again if his heart stops? Is my sister's love of cooking or safety more important? These are the sorts of decisions that death experts grapple with daily and that many of us will face, whether we are prepared or not.

This project started as a way of discovering what elder care workers had learned from their work. What sustains them? How do they manage working around death? Family caregivers like Janet Conroy learn about themselves, the person they care for, and the relationship with the person in their care. What do elder care workers learn, and how do they make sense of their work? I wanted to know how workers prevented depression and burnout and what motivated them to do their work. However, their accounts quickly altered my search for mere survival strategies. Instead of *surviving* this work, workers talked about loving their work, feeling called to it, experiencing pride because of it, and, like Janet Conroy, becoming bigger and better persons as a result of knowing the people in their care. So instead of survival strategies, I offer these, the most frequently cited lessons from the end of life. I believe that, like me, readers may benefit from hearing the insights of this group of workers.

Eight Lessons from the End of Life

Allison Stillwell frequently visits her mother, Sharon Stillwell, who lives at Winthrop House. In the first few years that Sharon lived there, she participated in many activities: she sang in a church choir, attended movie nights, helped lead sing-alongs in the care center, attended daily meals in the dining room, and volunteered at the local library. Now Sharon is eighty-four, aged beyond her years by a stroke in her eightieth year that took away her speech and all of her independent movement. She lives on, but her ability to make choices or participate in life is entirely dependent on the help of others. At times, it seems she reacts to music or the photos that Allison organizes into albums for her, but at other times, it is less clear what she understands. Seven months ago, she was put into hospice because her weight was dropping rapidly, her breathing seemed more difficult, and she appeared more withdrawn. Her placement in hospice signified that her family doctor estimated that Sharon had six or fewer months to live. Then, four months ago, during her third month in hospice care, she started to choke on the food that the nurses, nurse's aides, and her daughter gave her. The director of nursing, concerned about the choking hazard, asked Allison if it was okay to puree Sharon's food. Allison said yes.

In a month, Sharon's weight had gone back up, and as a result of what registers as a health improvement, she was forcibly removed from hospice. Now, four months later, Allison mourns her decision and its unforeseen consequences; her mother's body has rebounded, and now she will live longer with even more limited capacities but without the added care of hospice workers. Most of all, Allison regrets the uninformed role she played in her mother's improvement. She believes her mother is ready to die, but now she will live longer. Allison accidentally exacerbated the frail, frustrating, and increasingly powerless stage of her mother's life. Allison was faced with a choice: either puree her mother's food and prolong her life or give her solid food and accept that she will die from choking. Had she recognized the choice to puree the food for what it was, she would have said no, but she did not know what the likely outcome would be. For Allison and Sharon, this was one of the moments in the threshold between life and death. This decision elongated the dying process.

Being a death novice, Allison could not foresee the consequences of her choice. By contrast, elder care workers do know, intuitively and practically, many of the signposts and tendencies that characterize how we die now. At times, they struggle with how to reveal what they can foresee to their residents, but they often are able to anticipate and predict what death novices cannot. When I interviewed elder care nurses, nurse's aides, social workers, administrators, chaplains, and doctors, I was startled by how similar their concerns were. I had expected workers to be concerned about coping with death, but instead, I found that workers were grappling actively and sometimes frustratingly with these dilemmas of the threshold. The stress of their jobs did not come from the regular deaths of the elderly residents in their care. Rather, the workers' main stressor was witnessing residents make difficult decisions and have experiences that workers wished they could protect them from. The stressors for them, then, are the new conditions of old age and prolonged dying. As pioneers in this stage of life, elder care workers develop a set of priorities and beliefs regarding this time of life. Some of these "lessons" apply to the residents in their care, and some are lessons about life and death more generally. Taken together, these lessons are like navigational tools for the new social terrain unearthed by the longevity dividend. It is to these lessons I now turn.

Lesson One: Medical Technology Can Extend Life beyond All Sense

Medical care and technologies—both subtle and extreme—can prolong life but run the risk that life will continue in the absence of quality. Subtle interventions, such as pureeing food and offering antibiotics, as well as more extreme measures, such as breathing devices and hip replacements, work together to give older Americans more days, months, and years. But these medical interventions do not and cannot ensure quality of life. Medical ethicist Daniel Callahan refers to the notion of technological brinkmanship to capture the series of moral and practical dilemmas associated with the contemporary dying process. "The general problem was quickly identified well over two decades ago: since medical technology can prolong lives beyond the point of all sense and value, what can be done to avoid such a result?" (Callahan 1993: 37). When I interviewed Sara Shade, a onetime nurse who became a hospital administrator, she echoed Callahan's concern, explaining the challenge as "medicine that extends life beyond all reason." Scholars like Callahan and practitioners like Shade agree that alongside the many benefits of new technology come the challenges of prolonged dying, questions about quality of life, and many moments of both moral and practical ambiguity for participants.

In addition to the remarkable inheritance of longer lives, people face rapid changes in the life course, including worse health,

longer illnesses, slower deaths, longer aging, and increased dementia (Callahan 1993: 47). Because death now principally comes
from chronic and degenerative diseases of aging, the dying process
is characterized by a prolonged period of inconsistent decline in
which the dying person improves briefly, reaches what participants
call "a new normal," and then declines again. In an interview, physician Lisa Benstrom explained how chronic and degenerative illnesses often present the dying persons and their family members
with a series of changes like "stair steps" that go up and down,
eventually leading to death.

> With most illnesses—you figure your normal functioning
> is at a hundred, and you get ill and your functioning drops
> to sixty. And then it will come back up to seventy, but it
> won't go back to a hundred, and people aren't used to that
> stair-step sort of problem. So people think about a smooth
> decline, and there are good days and bad days, particularly
> with an illness like Parkinson's, but if you really want to
> know the quirks of the illness, you're going to need to take
> a big step back and look. I usually draw a stock-market sort
> of graph, and the stock is going down—if I'm talking to
> my neighbor or whatever, I draw it in the air. So, like, how
> long does it go? And you need to understand that it goes
> down.

Dying individuals and their loved ones often struggle to know
what these "stair-step" changes in health mean in terms of progno-
sis, duration of life remaining, and how to respond to each change
as it develops. Because chronic and degenerative diseases may
make the outer horizon of life difficult to ascertain, end-of-life
workers are often escorts through this ambiguous dying process,
helping patients and their families "read" the signs and interpret

the meanings of bodily changes and health challenges (Bern-Klug 2004). As Dr. Benstrom explains, family members are often so closely involved in the details of their elder relative's health status that they have trouble identifying patterns or even recognizing where they are in the trajectory of an illness. Workers can use death competence and accrued experience to help family members and residents make sense of the particular disease course. These workers are also often in a position to help families with the dilemmas related to technological brinkmanship, including the question of when medical interventions should be curtailed. Are there times when it is more loving to withhold treatments? These are some of the difficult questions surrounding how we die now.

Positioned as they are at the center of the possibilities from and limits of the longevity dividend, many end-of-life workers I interviewed expressed concern about what they view as the excessive focus on prolonging life. In fact, most had developed strong opinions about what qualifies as quality of life, what counts as a good death, and what is the role of medical interventions. They worried about how frequently elders were moved—often to a hospital—to receive medical treatment because such moves could be so difficult and even alarming for elders. Others worried that very few elders (or their family members) feel empowered to turn down medical treatments, no matter how extreme. Among the people I interviewed, there was a virtual consensus that the elders they served were at risk for excessive medical interventions. Their concern was strongly felt as a motivation to help elders navigate end-of-life decisions. It also influenced many of them to create personal plans for avoiding overtreatment when their own end comes. Workers were troubled that the availability of potentially life-extending medical technologies is often a distraction to family members. They related instances in which they thought that extreme medical treatments were accepted or embraced in the hope that death could be delayed or somehow avoided. Chaplain Mary Montour talked about helping family members think about dying directly rather than pinning all their hopes on life-prolonging technologies.

> I think it's insane the number of people whose families try to keep them alive. And it's, I think, based on the fear of death. Or the fear of saying good-bye. And that's another piece of it—why do we feel so strongly that good-bye is more than just that? Why do we feel like it has to be endless? I think the vast majority of my work is normalizing the end of life as well as death, and being able to celebrate it.

Chaplain Montour's comment that "I think it's insane the number of people whose families try to keep them alive" sounds harsh, maybe even cruel. Wouldn't it be insane *not* to extend a loved one's life if the means are available? Yet this sentiment is practically universal among the people I interviewed. What the families focus on is the long shot: the possibility of more time together. And it is not insane to want that. However, what workers like Montour see is the other end of the decision: how often death comes anyway, amid or immediately following a difficult and painful procedure. Even when the long shot works out and the resident's life is extended, they have witnessed the new challenges, pains, and losses that accompany such interventions. And finally, as Montour points out, many workers believe there is an opportunity cost—that families often pursue medical interventions in lieu of saying good-bye, acknowledging that the end is near, or taking the opportunity to celebrate the dying person's life. Chaplain Montour's focus on celebration may seem surprising initially, but it was a sentiment echoed by most of the workers I interviewed. For them, death is not the only thing to be avoided. Workers try to help family members come to grips with the reality of death so that they do not make choices, in an effort to avoid it, that they later regret.

Lesson Two: You Have Choices

Lack of experience with the dying process and faith in the seeming miracles offered by medical technology can combine to produce a deep denial that death is inevitable. Many family members, and occasionally the dying patient or resident, struggle with the faulty conviction that death is forever avoidable through increasingly heroic medical interventions. As Diana Rodriguez, a hospice administrator, explains, "It's very hard for Americans not to get caught up in our own rescue fantasies or the rescue fantasies of our providers." Like Rodriguez, many end-of-life workers must grapple with the rescue fantasies of patients, family members, and sometimes doctors or other medically trained staff. So one of the lessons that many workers feel they have learned from witnessing so many deaths is that the goal should be *better,* not longer, lives. Many workers want families to shift their focus away from heroics and the drama of "fighting" illness; they would prefer to escort families through that threshold time in a more peaceful and deliberate way. Workers tell horror stories that function as cautionary tales about residents who were encouraged to fight desperately against their own mortality. Rodriguez describes it as the "relentless pursuit of life at any quality."

For many workers, it seems that death competence can take the form of death acceptance. They claim that denial and anxiety are reduced through repeated contact with death. As Eva Crowley, a hospice nurse, explains, older people are also less likely to deny death's inevitability because of their own experiences with losing loved ones and friends.

I think a lot of people are in denial. Not everyone . . . but I guess that's why I like working with the elderly, because they're less in denial. But, you know, it's natural for older people to be coming to grips with it, because they've had more experience with it than someone young.

Implicit in Crowley's comment is a view that many workers convey: often the family and friends, not the dying person, are the ones who are seeking more time at any cost. Many workers said that by focusing on more time, families missed opportunities to be present in the dying process. To take the threshold concept further, workers observed that family members focused backward, toward the room of living into which their loved one could not reenter, and in that focus, they missed out on participating in the threshold itself—when life is wrapping up and moving toward death.

End-of-life workers describe denial as an unfortunate stance toward death because it does not allow patients, residents, or their family members the opportunity to engage meaningfully with the dying process. Denial, for them, ensures that death will be encountered as a crisis rather than a process, with time for communication and opportunity for choice. Instead, many practitioners believe that some knowledge about the dying process can help family members communicate clearly with one another and make confident decisions even in the shadow of mortality. As Crowley explains, "Everyone is going to die and leave this world, and health care is not going to change that. We're all going to die, but we have choices in how we want to do it." Her notion of choice—of having choices—was central to many workers' views of the dying process. In this view, residents and family members could not control death, but they still had choices that could affect the time leading up to death, including whether or not to pursue medical interventions and what attitude or posture they would assume toward death. As many of the stories here show, such choices arise again and again during the twists and turns of prolonged dying. Throughout the "stair steps"—the ups and downs—residents and family members have to make many decisions, large and small, about what stance they are going to take toward death's approach.

Most workers were explicit about their desire to ease dying residents, and particularly their families, into the pursuit of meaningful exchange and living in the time remaining, replacing the relentless pursuit of more time with a focus on quality of life and respect, even *reverence,* for the cycle of life. Helping families shift their focus during prolonged dying processes also becomes a subject for training. Dr. Suzy Hoefield talks about how she trains gerontology interns to recognize opportunities in the dying process.

> [I train them to] look at a person holistically and also to respect the cycle of life. That's how we have to deal with the elderly. It's *okay* for someone to die; we're all gonna do it, you know. And as I taught my [students] in the facilities, if that person dies comfortably, with dignity, and preferably with people who love them around them, then that's a good thing to think about.

Similarly, hospital administrator Sara Shade encourages the nurses and nurse's aides she trains to help families recognize and facilitate the dying process rather than fight it.

> I would hope [that my trainees would be] much more pragmatic about the process of death. After a point, there's no way you can stop it. When there's no way to stop it, it doesn't help the patient to dig your heels in and, you know, beg them to live, and, I mean, I've seen that. Patients . . . so thoroughly exhausted. And the families crying, holding

their hand. "Please, you've got to hang on, Forest. You've got to hang on." For what? To send a loved one out the door? 'Cause then they have the guilt of letting down the family, but then they need to. They need to be released to go.

Shade's frustration is evident in her description. She is recalling patients for whom longer lives were *worse* than dying. Talking with workers, I began to see that they were forced to moralize and take positions on the difficult decisions that new medical technologies had produced. Sometimes, as in the case of Sharon Stillwell, the intervention seems mundane—pureeing food—when it is actually dramatic: elongating life for months. At other times, the intervention is major, such as a hip replacement or open-heart surgery. In all these cases, residents and family members do not always recognize that they have a choice. Workers see it as one of their goals to help families recognize options, particularly the option of intentionally letting go, which includes declining some available treatments and openly acknowledging, even *welcoming*, death's approach.

Lesson Three: Fear a Bad Death, Not Death Itself

End-of-life workers develop strong opinions about when longer lives become worse lives. These workers are firm advocates for the possibilities for quality at the end of life but are also mindful of the attendant risk that quality can be compromised by medical measures. They refer to both risks and benefits as they try to gently prepare elders to make choices in keeping with their own values and commitments. For example, social worker Rita Sanford explains that she helps residents imagine how their death can have meaning for them.

They're coming here [Winthrop House], day one, and the doctor's saying, "Consider hospice," so then that starts the clock. But then I think the majority of those who know it's their final stop want to talk about it, and they'll tell you what they want. You know, "I want to go to bed after having a great day and I don't want to wake up." And they talk about the "pleasant" death. "I want to be like so-and-so, who was at supper that night, and then she died." And the residents actually are *very* clear about that. It's the families who may be doing that for the first time.

Rita describes her job as one of bridging the divide between residents' and their families' perceived competence and preparation. Like Rita, many elder care workers recalled family members who resisted death or fought the dying process. These comments reveal an unstated vision of a "good" death that is shared by many workers. Hospice has an official definition of a good death that includes saying good-bye, asking for forgiveness, forgiving others, and having some say in how one's life ends. By contrast, elder care facilities do not have a set notion of a good death, but given the commonalities in workers' accounts of undesirable deaths, the basic contours of a belief system take shape. On the basis of their frequent encounters with death, the vast majority of workers believe that bad deaths occur when the family rails against the dying process, when the dying person is for some reason unable to express his or her final wishes, or when fears get in the way of intentional leave-taking.

According to Sara Shade, the fear of death actually comes from two sources: "fear of the unknown and fear of pain." She considers it her job to help patients understand and manage pain and subsequently escape that fear. "The unknown cannot be resolved, but I can help with the pain." The connections between fear of death and fear of pain also turned up in K. E. Steinhauser, E. C. Clipp, and M. McNeilly's (2000: 828) study: "Many focus group participants feared dying in pain. Portrayals of bad deaths usually mentioned inadequate analgesia during cure-directed therapies that were perceived as too aggressive." Scholars call these fears "anticipatory fears" (Steinhauser, Clipp, and McNeilly 2000). These fears are often fed by a lack of knowledge about how death really happens, so death experts can aid in easing anticipatory fear by educating dying individuals and their families about the context of contemporary dying processes, including how pain is managed, stages they can anticipate, choices they may need to make, and factors they may want to consider in their decision making.

Elder care workers understandably focus on what is controllable: they cannot vanquish death, but they can help with pain and outlook. In most workers' view, bad dying was characterized by lack of opportunity to plan ahead, arrange personal affairs, decrease family burden, or say good-bye. Ira Byock, a physician and something of a guru on dying, describes dying persons' fears in similar terms.

> People fear tangible things related to when and how they will eventually die: being abandoned; becoming undignified in terms of what they do, how they look, and how they smell; being a burden to their families—not only a physical strain, but also a financial hardship; dying in pain. (Byock 1997: 241)

Being around death, workers and many residents start to envision what they want at the time of their own death and, perhaps more importantly, what they do not want. The redundancy of these visions is important because the fears that accompany them are avoidable. Residents crack jokes about dying in one's sleep because most, if not all, of the residents hope for such a quick and painless end. But workers and residents in elder care facilities recognize that slow declines are more common than fast endings. Being unable to pick between sudden and prolonged dying, residents receive help from workers to control what they can about the circumstances of their end.

Lesson Four: You Can See Death Coming

As death novices, we encounter death as a mystery the first time, usually through the death of a close family member or friend. Death seems unpredictable, unwieldy, and most of all frightening. But for end-of-life workers, the dying process starts to take on a recognizable shape and have identifiable steps. In an elder community, dying is routine, even mundane. Dying is important, but it is not surprising. And finally, dying is often accompanied by specific signposts.

Workers look for specific signs indicating when the active dying process has begun. Here are some of the most common ones that workers identified in interviews:

- Residents show less interest in details about the wider world: sports scores, weather, the menu, the date, and the news.
- Days, even weeks, prior to death, residents show declining interest in eating.
- Residents often begin to talk about going on a journey.
- Even among those who have been withdrawn for a long time, moments of clarity or clear speech—often brief—may occur. Some call these "awakenings."
- Toes may curl.

- Knees and lower legs may mottle and start to spot.
- As the circulation of blood weakens, the extremities begin to feel cool. The skin may lose some of its ruddiness, turning grayish or bluish.
- Long after losing interest in food, residents may lose their sense of thirst and thus any interest in drinking even water.
- Shortly before death, residents may develop what workers call a "death rattle." This is a cracking sound in the throat that can be alarming for loved ones and caregivers. As residents lose the ability or focus to clear saliva from the airway, the saliva rattles in the throat.
- Residents may reach up and out.
- Breathing may become much slower, signaling the decrease of circulation in the respiratory center. Sometimes the breathing may even seem to stop, and very quiet sighs may follow, until the breath finally ends.

Knowing these signs and helping family and friends recognize them help remove the surprise of death and the shock of mortality. Death comes in recognizable steps rather than in unprecedented, frightening changes. By marking these signposts, end-of-life workers can help family members intentionally approach the death of their loved one, step by step.

For residents and family members, the open acknowledgment of the dying process and information about how death *tends* to happen can be uncomfortable, or it can be a welcome release from the denial of death. Speaking about the process of her mother's dying, Janet Conroy describes how liberating knowledge shared by end-of-life workers was for her.

And [elder care nurses were] the ones who told me. . . . Even the nursing staff on the behavioral unit never told me what happens when somebody stops eating—what does that mean and how do you make these choices—because they're still all about medical intervention. So once I finally was able to talk to the [elder care workers], I was like, "How do I even make these decisions?" And they were like, "That's very common, and this is what happens if that's the route that your mother's body is following." And I was like, "Well, that makes perfect sense, doesn't it?"

For some dying individuals and their family members, embracing and expanding on the death competence of experienced end-of-life workers offer a possibility of greeting dying with more than fear and uncertainty.

Workers also reported using these signs of death's approach to discourage family members from putting pressure on dying persons to "stay longer." Many workers I interviewed reported witnessing dying residents "holding on" for a particular purpose. Residents waited to see a beloved daughter return home from overseas, to be in attendance at a wedding, or to learn that a grandchild was born. As Ira Byock explains, dying persons "often exhibit an uncanny control over the timing of death" (1997: 225). Sara Shade describes witnessing these events.

You know, we've seen patients that [we] did not think were gonna live to the end of this shift. But somewhere, midway, we heard that such-and-such's son is gonna be here from California tomorrow afternoon. And then the patient stays around until tomorrow afternoon, and sees the son, and then dies a few hours later.

These acts of will and control in the very weak and dying convinced many workers that family members could turn a good death bad through undue pressure. In short, workers had organized the death process by identifying likely signposts, and they then conveyed the signposts as part of their work in helping families see and make choices in that threshold between life and death.

Lesson Five: You Can Plan on Death

End-of-life workers count on death. They plan for it in their own lives, and they hope that their residents and patients will do the same. Chaplain Phyllis Star makes a case for the value of planning, calling herself a control monger.

> *Any* state of transition in life—diminishing health, moving to a retirement community, dying . . . the fear that comes from being unprepared, to me, is much greater than a fear of knowing what I'm feeling. And the more [of a] control freak you are, then the more valuable it is to you to be in control of your life and run for it, rather than have it suddenly hit you in the face.

For Star, death can be encountered either as a crisis or as a predictable stage, like other stages in life. To her, making plans offers an antidote to fearing death. The chaplain also names a tendency that runs through workers' outlooks: control in the face of death is good. And most workers agree with Star that control is not only good but also achievable. So while death cannot be delayed, it can be partially controlled through careful planning.

All of the people I interviewed—*every single worker*—spoke about the need to make plans for death. Dr. Suzy Hoefield explains that she no longer fears death but rather fears avoidance of death.

Death is just the natural progression of life. And if you're thinking about, if you're worried about loss of function or loss of independence, do something *now,* to make a *difference*! Keep yourself in better shape, make appointments for support in your older years. You know, if you think your plan is going in a nursing home, well then, make *arrangements.*

Like Star and Hoefield, the workers believe that making plans is possible, preferable, and powerful. For them, dying is a foreseeable stage of life, like adolescence, and it is improved by planning, just like having a college fund. Their views were so consistent on this point that it seemed to me that fear had been replaced with a mandate to plan. Their awareness of the twists and turns that could accompany prolonged dying had made them advocates for planning. This belief in planning—almost an orthodoxy—combined with faith in the power of choice and control. To lay down plans before death begins is to acknowledge its inevitability, to envision better and worse pathways to death, and to feel empowered to exert one's will today into the future. For workers, their work had taught them that unplanned deaths gave them fewer opportunities to play out a resident's wishes. The question remains whether this sense of control is illusory or not. Many studies show that advance directives are often ignored in emergency situations. Despite this, if a nursing home resident communicates plans to long-term staff and family and manages to die in that place, rather than in a hospital or ambulance, those plans may succeed in operating as effective directives to those who accompany them through death.

Given their conviction that planning on death was so important, I started asking the people I was interviewing if *they* had made plans for their own end. Forty-eight out of fifty had done so.

Planning was not simply a mantra of advice to residents but also one that the workers had internalized and followed for themselves. For example, Clark Daily, who runs the food service at Winthrop House, explains his thinking about his own plans.

> One of the things I did maybe six years ago was I made sure I had my own will. You know, I was single, in my forties. I thought—I want to make sure things end up the way I want them. Because things happen to people my age. I think, being in this [line of work] you have a different outlook—you're not going to be so careless about it. You have a different outlook on life and what's important. So I wanted those things in place. Because I recently have seen both sides of the spectrum within long-term care: it can be a wonderful experience, and it can be horrible. And I didn't want it to be horrible. And, also, I think everybody has a responsibility for your family, or loved ones, whoever you're connected with. And a lot of people don't do that. And they don't *think* about it. I don't know if it's just the *American* people—we don't think about our mortality—until it's too late.

Daily's work has brought him into close contact with people whom he views as dying well and dying poorly. He sees putting plans in place as one tool at his disposal to exercise some control over his own end. His readiness to make plans is a result of his work, which has changed how he thinks about living and dying.

> [This work] sensitizes you to the things many people give up. Between now and the end of my life, in my mind, is about thirty-five years. So I see myself living in a nursing facility somewhere at the end of my life. And whenever I

share that with people, they almost freak, because most people can't imagine that. It doesn't scare me—I don't want to die alone; I don't want to be in physical need and therefore maybe in mental need. I want to be there with people who know me. And I know that happens. And the value of having support, having people whose work is to be with you and to be trained to be with you as you go through the end of life—I understand that in a way that I didn't before.

Just as one anticipates children growing older, the arrival of midlife, or the need to replace a roof every ten years or so, workers like Daily make plans for death. Doing so makes them feel comfortable and ready. Their goal is to encourage the residents they come into contact with to do the same. When Daily talks about his plans, he also talks about a vision he has of how he might die—his planning is designed to increase the odds that he will have that experience. As I listened to one worker after another share such a vision, I realized that this was one of the side effects of the work. Having witnessed a range of deaths encouraged them to think about their own. Their visions are elaborate, detailed, and, in almost all cases, written down. Planning on death seemed to be a way that workers have reconciled the frequent deaths they observe and the inevitability of their own end.

Lesson Six: Small Acts Matter

Even for families who have put plans in place, family members and friends often still struggle with what to do when active dying begins. Unlike with sudden deaths, prolonged dying takes some time. The threshold combines aspects of living with aspects of dying, which can confuse participants. On this front too, family members and friends often turn to end-of-life workers for expertise and modeling.

Elder care workers assist by observing, tracking, understanding, responding to, and communicating changes in the body and routines of the residents they serve. When it comes time to help her residents die, or help family members of the resident deal with their loved one's death, a nurse's aide named Bristol Olson relies on her embodied, routine knowledge of the resident to provide care.

> You are doing something that not a lot of people can handle, that not a lot of people can do. And you are that person; I mean, when you are elderly, the family only comes once a week. And you are there. You are the one that tells them good night every single night. You are the one that bathes them. You *know* them better than the family does now. You kiss Margaret good night every night.

In the face of others' dying, Bristol continues to do something for the residents in her care: she communicates her consistent concern through care of their bodies and through her affection. In doing so, she models what end-of-life workers say is so hard for many people in the face of death: to continue doing things for the dying person. One resident likes to have a washcloth on her forehead, another feels better with an extra dash of powder, another likes his feet rubbed when Bristol or another nurse's aide has time on her shift. Bristol's expertise, her competence around dying, comes from recognizing and remembering what helps her residents to feel more comfortable and therefore less afraid. Many elder care workers like Bristol also have to encourage family members to touch and talk to their loved one as they usually would because in the face of death some people become immobilized.

Family members struggle with the intimacy and messiness of

death. Recognizing changes, they often view dying as a reason to suspend normalcy and, intentionally or not, distance themselves from the dying person. Relatives and friends also worry about transgressing old boundaries when they do care work that involves nakedness, touch, or new dependencies. For many family members, the loved one's new status of actively dying confuses them. This death might be a first or one of few for them. Relatives may feel they should treat the dying person delicately or may even believe that dying is sacred and unlike other parts of life. By contrast, most workers believe that sustaining routines can be a crucial form of communication.

From the perspective of the elder care workers I interviewed, too often family members are intimidated by these changes and fail to touch and take care of their loved one at their own peril. These workers believe that small acts matter and that doing something is the only thing left before death. They observe that family members freeze up and avoid the dying person as if by refusing to acknowledge the new needs and changes in their loved one's body, death might be avoided. But these caring tasks are some of the only interactions possible in the final days and weeks of life for many people. As Sara Shade explains, family members need to be encouraged to overcome their fears and feelings of futility to stay connected.

> [I tell them] don't be afraid to touch them. After everything, don't be afraid to touch them. You can hold them; you can kiss them; you can hug them. And some people are afraid if somebody's getting ready to die, and it becomes obvious that they're afraid to touch them.

So elder care workers encourage family members to pick up a washcloth, to rub a back, to hold a hand, to brush Mom's hair, to wet Dad's lips, because these simple acts are a form of contact and connection in the days or hours before death parts them.

Many workers expressed concerns that because deaths in pop culture are often dramatic—marked by violence, dying confessions, or revealed secrets—families sometimes seemed to wait for additional signs that the end was coming. Workers described what they saw as missed opportunities to offer small acts of kindness to the dying person as a result of waiting for a sign that never came. While there was nothing particularly sacred or striking about pulling up the covers, turning on a fan, or feeding ice chips, in workers' minds, attending to these needs represented the remaining opportunities for friends and family to express regard and love. Scholar Julia Twigg describes the quiet centrality of daily customs to sustaining identity and connection.

> Activities like bathing and washing play a central part in domestic life. . . . Getting up, dressing, eating, sleeping, excreting provide the bedrock of social existence. These activities, however, exist at a level that is rarely brought into conscious articulation or review; indeed in modern Western societies we are largely educated to ignore them, regarding them as too trivial or too private for comment. But such activities offer a rich source of implicit meaning in people's lives, sustaining and expressing relationships, endorsing values and beliefs, providing an existential coherence to individuals' lives. (2000: 4)

Family members may refrain from helping with these daily rituals because such support is often relegated to the lowest-status workers in elder care facilities, such as nurse's aides and housekeeping staff. Yet these rituals are the final pillars of "being someone" in the face of death. For example, social worker Rita Sanford describes how nurse's aides often become the primary source of information about daily habits and changes for elders in nursing care.

> The CNAs are doing the day-to-day tasks. They know what time they have to go to bed, their ritual after supper, dental care, their dentures, so they have that type of relationship of trust with that resident, but then it also carries over to the family. When the family comes over on a Saturday at two o'clock, they know to go to Bristol and say, "How's Dad today?" And she would know, you know, if he had a rough night last night.

Workers believe that daily rituals sustain the dying and that helping with these rituals is a way of being with the dying person, of communicating compassion and understanding, and, finally, of paying attention and respect to them in their final days and hours. This belief is a way of valuing labor that is largely invisible. To the family member who is paralyzed by the thought of losing a loved one, workers say, "Do something," and in doing so, they avoid saying, "Do what I do. Take care of their bodies, sustain their routines." Their advice for how to break the paralysis that fear can induce is to labor in the time preceding death.

Lesson Seven: It Is Never Too Late to Say What You Mean

Workers believe that, in addition to touching a dying person, speaking frankly with the dying person and with the other people connected to him or her is crucial. Elder care workers encourage family members to communicate throughout the process of dying: from diagnosis to the last breath. They witness family members and friends make several errors in communicating: they turn on one another, they fall silent, they internalize their grief, and they

miss opportunities to say what they mean. As one of the physicians I interviewed, Dr. E. J. Robbinson, explains, many death
novices react to their awareness of death's approach with silence
rather than conversation.

> All of a sudden you're going to the hospital and . . . you're
> gonna *die,* and you say to your doctor, "Well, yeah, I've
> had this cancer for five months. You didn't tell me!" And
> many people try to "protect" their loved ones. And that is
> also a big myth. You don't protect anybody by doing that.
> And so one of the things that we try for in the inner family
> is to help people communicate. Communication skills—to
> get people to say things that they're feeling, you know, in a
> protected environment that they can say these things.

As Dr. Robbinson points out, death is not successfully avoided by
silence. Many end-of-life workers I interviewed believe that communication should be enlivened and heightened during the dying
process because, after all, as death approaches, the opportunities
to communicate decrease incrementally.

Workers expressed the view that dying persons are often the
most aware of their near future—they know they are dying and
can benefit from frank talk and honest conclusions with loved
ones. But too often, friends and family dance around the fact
that someone is dying—focusing on more time, hope for cures,
or minutiae. In the process, rare and fleeting opportunities to be
honest with one another and to say good-bye, offer apologies and
forgiveness when needed, and communicate one's true feelings are
squandered.

End-of-life workers try to encourage friends and family to stay
attuned to the process and to speak to the dying person. As death
approaches, hearing is arguably the last possibility for connec-

tion. Studies suggest that hearing continues long after the other senses shut down, so even after the opportunity to do something has passed, the opportunity to say something continues. Yet many family members begin to talk *about* the dying person rather than to the dying person. Sara Shade describes the recent death of a woman whose family members stayed focused and continued to talk frankly with her.

> It's hard to know what the family needs at a specific time. I try to read people, you know. I actually think intuition, in terms of interacting with people, plays a big role in how effective you are in facilitating the situation for them. The whole death process, there's so much that is nebulous; you can't just say, "This is the deal." You know, you can't do that. There are some general *guidelines.* . . . You try to make the patients comfortable and ease them out in a manageable mood. You know, not crazy chaotic, stressful, so that they have some peace of mind. A calm situation: it is possible! The lady that we had fairly recently, she [passed well]. Her family was at the bedside, and everybody was up, and she was crying. And they were calm, and they talked to her. And that's one of the things *I* try to tell people is— keep talking to them, they can *hear* you. Hearing seems to be the last thing to go. Keep talking.

As Shade explains, talking is one way that family and friends can accompany the people they love into death itself. Given the delicacy of people's emotions, it seems that workers mainly *model* continuous communication rather than become heavy-handed with their advice. Particularly low-level workers do not feel empowered to tell families to talk. Rather, like Shade, they admire families who manage to keep talking to the end.

Lesson Eight: Accompanying Others through Death Is a Privilege

The final "lesson" that emerged in talking with workers was that helping others die is not a burden—it is a privilege. Of the fifty individuals I interviewed who have ushered someone else toward death, the most common refrain was *gratitude* for the opportunity. As a researcher, I was caught off guard by this finding. More than half of the participants directly expressed gratitude, saying that it was an honor or that they felt lucky to be involved in the dying process. At first I was surprised by this response to what seemed to me to be very challenging work, but over time I came to expect it because so many workers conveyed gratitude for the opportunity to be with residents and their families at a difficult and also important time. I wanted to know more about what made these workers feel grateful. When I probed participants' answers, I came to recognize three reasons for the gratitude: overcoming fear, living more fully, and being engaged in meaningful work. So this final lesson is not a directive or a sign to look for; instead, it is about what workers believe is *possible* as a result of witnessing many deaths and developing death competence.

First, daily or weekly contact with death provided end-of-life workers an opportunity to engage with their own fears of death. Over time, elder care workers felt that their ability to manage the pain, grief, fear, and confusion that can accompany death improved and that they were stronger as a result.

Second, by overcoming the paralyzing fear of death, they felt more alive. Overall, their experiences with dying have changed them by making them more communicative and more willing to touch others, speak frankly, and make plans for their own lives. Consequently, they felt more secure and found their days more rewarding. Sara Shade describes how she has changed as a result of her work.

> Myself, personally, I think I've gathered a whole lot more life experiences, and I myself am more comfortable with death. So I don't have the same kind of anxiety that I used to have. I mean, I can tell a real difference in the way that I approach it, and I really try to be more therapeutic for the family members who are left than I could have been before.

In short, the routine engagement with death was transformative for workers precisely because it was difficult and rare. This work set them apart, and it made them feel awake and alive to all of life's changes. The continuing presence of death was also a reminder of the preciousness of life. Hospice nurse Eva Crowley demonstrates this sense of heightened awareness when she describes how she'll approach her own death: "When my time comes, I'll just stock my freezer up with Häagen-Dazs, put in a margarita machine, and enjoy the end." Workers express confidence, even bravado, in the face of death.

Finally, death competence and the changes that accompanied its development made workers proud. Workers across the occupational spectrum feel proud of doing work that makes use of so many of their skills and abilities. They view their work as demanding and worthy of great effort. End-of-life workers felt honored when they feel meaningfully engaged in other people's dying processes. Administrator Diana Rodriguez, described it as reaping the rewards of "grief work" (Kübler-Ross 1969; Callahan 1993). This intentional movement through the pain wrought by mortality is described not only as hard won—the result of practice—but also as a very important type of work, which they feel grateful to be involved in providing.

When workers nudge residents or relatives to embrace the dying process, they do so partly because of their own transformation resulting from their engagement with death. In encouraging, sometimes maybe even *directing*, family members to actively engage with dying, they are sharing an approach to death that they think is preferable to denial and avoidance. Their advice to pursue an intentional, sustained process of ushering another person into death reflects their own values and arises from the perceived rewards that their own work with death has provided.

Strategies and Rewards

It is important to note that all of the guiding principles workers subscribe to not only provide them with confidence and grounding but also lend them some control over their working conditions. First, using death competence to structure how they help others deal with upcoming deaths makes their work easier. Death competence provides workers with signposts to point out to new families, residents, and patients whom they encounter. By correctly anticipating likely moments or experiences that the family will encounter, end-of-life workers gain credibility, and their account of death and counsel on what to expect carry more authority. Patients, residents, and the residents' family members feel assisted toward death, and because they do, end-of-life workers feel as though they have done their job well.

By providing a template within which families can seek to make sense of individual dying experiences, end-of-life workers educate patients and their families about the dying process while also gaining control over their work process by explaining, and therefore shaping, the dying experience before it is completed.

As such, death competence can serve both the patients and the organizational imperatives. Workers can facilitate the needs of the dying while also ensuring the smooth functioning of the organization by anticipating and smoothing out potential obstacles, such as complaints, outbursts, resistance, or danger for participants. Since continuing care retirement communities operate in a litigious and regulatory context, some choices by workers may also address institutional needs to follow regulations, observe protocol, avoid lawsuits, or keep residents happy. Any or all of these motivations might combine at one time or another, but each addresses a way in which competence makes workers better at their jobs.

There are risks to death competence. One is that the approach that workers advocate will become so solidified that alternative approaches will be difficult to pursue on their watch. Given the common base of beliefs informing the decisions of long-term workers at Winthrop House, their experiences and subsequent commitments form a kind of template that encourages one way of approaching death while implicitly discouraging others. A related risk is that for some families, denial, silence, or distance might be necessary or even more useful, and for those families, help and accompaniment might be less forthcoming.

Despite these risks, an organized approach to actively engaging death makes sense because how we die now is frustrating, scary, and relatively unprecedented. The work that these people do is incredibly difficult. It is difficult like other service jobs that require workers to negotiate the needs of others, but these negotiations involve high stakes because they are final negotiations, entailing final wishes and final conversations. Being on the frontlines of prolonged dying is frightening because our longer lives deliver us slowly into death and new technologies offer up questions for which there are no "right" answers. So workers develop a set of approaches that make sense to them and that feel satisfying.

Director of nursing Tanya Santoro says, "We laugh every day. We have to; otherwise this work would [kill us]." Living and working in the constant shadow of death make workers painfully aware of the ins and outs of contemporary dying and how much is beyond the control of the dying persons, their doctors, nurses, aides, and loved ones. Sometimes workers have to laugh, and sometimes they end up feeling proud not of conquering death but of *meeting* it, day after day.

The main frustration shared by the people I interviewed is that avoiding death robs participants of the *rewards* of accompanying someone toward death. Such rewards were recounted previously in the story of Janet Conroy, who overcame her existential loneliness by ushering her mother into death. Like Janet, workers are convinced that being with someone in an intentional way as he or she approaches death is rewarding and transformative. In fact, reflecting on her own now-famous study of dying, Elisabeth Kübler-Ross expressed a similar sentiment. When asked if it was depressing to work with the dying, she responded that her work had made her appreciate every new day, increasing her awareness of the privilege of living. Similarly, the workers I interviewed believe that accompanying another person toward death is a privilege that should be embraced, not avoided. So when end-of-life workers rail against the denial of death, it is because they think that denying death risks missing out on the privilege of helping others die. Their stance is important because it is a vanguard engagement with death in a country that is getting older fast. The competence these workers share is an invitation to engage: an opportunity for the residents in their care and the rest of us as we move inexorably closer to our own mortal end.

5

Mutual Interdependency

Belonging, Recognition, and the Rewards of Caring for One Another

In the spring of 2012, I walked the streets, alleys, and sidewalks of Winthrop House to distribute my survey to residents. I carried my five-month-old son in a carrier on my chest. So when residents came to their door, they saw the face of a smiling baby, an unusual sight around campus. In one home, we sat down for a chat with a resident named Charlie Rothman. Charlie, in his seventies, talked about retirement and how much harder it has been for him to leave his profession than for his wife to adjust to retired life. "I'm lonely," he said.

Next door, I talked to Michael Corcoran. He had just returned from recycling the bottles and cans from his ninetieth birthday party. Amid reporting on his fabulous party to which over two hundred people came, he expressed concern about my father's recent death. When I asked Michael how he was doing, he said he had lost a daughter to cancer since I last saw him. We exchanged condolences and then talked more about his party.

Just down the block, we sat for a while with Mildred Hassidy, in her nineties, whose husband, Stan, is in much worse shape than she. Mildred lives in an apartment; Stan lives in the care center. She told me that she adds to his obituary every day—remembering some service he provided or an organization he led—to make sure that the record of his life is accurate. She said, "I have done my mourning." She views Stan as already gone; the man who remains today is not the man she remembers or mourns.

There is a lot of talk about wisdom at the end of life. As a social scientist, I am always suspicious of claims about wisdom for this reason: if we all fear the changes and inevitable declines of our bodies, then isn't it comforting to imagine that at least we also become inevitably smarter or, better yet, even wise? A comforting notion but unlikely, right? The hope that age would somehow transform all of us, making us better versions of ourselves in terms of identity and insight, even as the sand of our bodies, our earthly vessels, shifts beneath us is wishful but not necessarily true.[1]

Yet what I find at Winthrop House challenges my suspicion. I still do not believe that arriving at old age *necessarily* produces knowledge, but among many Winthrop House residents, I find what I think of as a kind of *deepening.* The elders I meet are more themselves, and they are also more present, more real than many young people. Wisdom does not spring from people at a certain age; they are still entirely themselves, and as such, some are smart, some are sharp, some are wise, and some are not. However, it seems to me that years of life toughen and reveal simultaneously. The toughening is like a kind of callus that forms from having lived many years. Michael Corcoran demonstrates this: even a remarkable, painful death like that of his child is one of many deaths he has witnessed. For Michael, death and life go hand in

---

1. Recent research has revealed biological evidence that maturity alters the brain in positive ways (Nuland 1993: 56).

hand: a funeral and a party. One does not make it to ninety years of age without seeing many deaths, even though some, like his daughter's, are out of order, or so it seems. So there is less drama, less surprise, and something that sounds (at least to someone like me who is younger and less seasoned) like clarity. The calluses of many years do not make for callous persons but rather produce clear persons: these things happen, even awful things, such as losing a daughter.

The passing of many years also provides revelations. In my time at Winthrop House, I came to expect frank talk and even revelations, like Mildred's admission that her grieving is complete and Charlie's that he is lonely. I learned to anticipate an almost complete lack of pretense. For instance, a resident named Margaret Clairis saw me for the first time after the birth of my son and said, "Isn't it amazing they come out of your body?" Conversation is marked by a kind of clarity that is at first quite intimidating because it is so contrary to the layers of pretense, performance, and distraction that accompany so many other interactions in daily life. No hollow civilities, no "happy weekend," no wasted breath. At Winthrop House people talk about what is actually going on: about what it is to be old in a society that does not value elders, about one's relationship to stuff, about family dynamics, about what people get paid and what they *should* get paid, about beliefs regarding the afterlife, and about the limits of love and the body. Intimidating indeed, but refreshing. I am not associating this frankness with old age; I think it is wrong to do so. I think plenty of elderly people, including some who live at Winthrop House, are angry, frustrated, fed up, and bottled up—nearly uncommunicative. I do not think old age inspires frankness necessarily, but it can, and something about this place makes that the norm here, in ways that are in direct contrast to what occurs in the bakery down the street, the school next door, and, I would argue, even some religious establishments. Here, people say what they mean, even when it is about a hurt—for example, "My husband is already gone" or "I am lonely."

In retrospect, I realize that when my students and I first started this research, we approached aging as a social problem and therefore viewed elders as people burdened by their old age. Doing this research has absolutely reversed that logic for me. Don't get me wrong—I am not saying that getting older is purely awesome: it is not. When one's body starts to change—not with the promise of youth but with the new limits of old age—it is tough, and there is no way around it. On top of that, friends, lovers, neighbors, and relatives die. The longer we live, the more people we bury. Aging is not without its costs; encountering limits and losing loved ones are the two main sources of sadness and struggle for elders. But what I expected to find and did not was a kind of dancing around the fact of old age. I liken it to going to the hospital with a sick person and resorting to euphemisms so as not to talk about the illness, the time that is left, or the parts of the body affected. In addition, I think my students and I thought we were going to need to keep the "secret" of their old age from residents. Naive indeed. Age and the fact of death come up in almost every conversation here, not in macabre or sad ways but rather in frank and clear ways. As Ron Peattie says, residents crack jokes about not wanting to buy six green bananas in case they do not live long enough to see the bananas ripen. At Winthrop House, residents are actively living out the longevity dividend, and they know that when they are dying, they will be sustained by the interdependent community to which they contributed and on which they rely.

As the previous chapters have demonstrated, the context in which we live out our longer lives matters a great deal, and facing the dilemmas of the threshold between life and death becomes more manageable when old age takes place within a community of care. In this final chapter, I presume that if an institution like Winthrop House can provide a context in which participants feel valued, connected, and even rewarded in the final years and days of life, then some of what works well in that institutional context may be transportable to the larger scene for elder care.

The most salient difference between Winthrop House and the larger society that surrounds it is the mutual *recognition* that Simone de Beauvoir describes in this way: "If we do not know what we are going to be, we cannot know what we are: Let us recognize ourselves in this old man and this old woman. It must be done if we are to take upon ourselves the entirety of our own human state" (1970: 12). Residents of Winthrop House recognize one another as an age cohort and as fellow sojourners in the "unknown country of old age" that the longevity dividend provides (Pipher 1999). They are living out old ages unlike those experienced by their own parents and grandparents, and they are actively learning from one another as they go. What's more, the community of Winthrop House defies the generational segregation that characterizes so much of American culture because staff members also recognize residents as partners on a similar journey. In this final chapter, I make a case for a broader practice of interdependency that will require offering recognition across generations and will encourage individuals of all ages to embrace the human capacities we contribute and the needs we develop across the life span. I posit that developing a practice of interdependency will require us to rethink care and dependency so that we approach the caregiving of our elders with the same patience and generosity we extend to children and infants. Doing so will enliven our awareness of a cycle of care in which we are already involved. The practice of interdependency requires us to anticipate and embrace dependency in later years, as we do in the early years of life, and to value the labor of caring for elders. Here, I offer some final suggestions based on my research at

Winthrop House, and I make a case for interdependency as a way of thinking and behaving that might allow for a move away from a cowardly approach to the end of life to one characterized by courage and connection.

Embracing Interdependency at the End of Life

As Mary Pipher explains, interdependency is a way of acknowledging a cycle of care and support that continues throughout the life course.

> At certain stages we are caretakers, at other stages we are cared for. Neither stage is superior to the other. Neither implies pathology or weakness. Both are just the results of life having seasons and circumstances. In fact, good mental health is not a matter of being dependent or independent, but of being able to accept the stage one is in with grace and dignity. It's an awareness of being, over the course of one's lifetime, continually interdependent. (1999: 52)

Interdependency frees up the energy, skills, and resources within generations to allow for intergenerational exchange that makes use of the abilities and addresses the needs of each individual. As feminist writer Audre Lorde points out, the generation gap puts a stranglehold on knowledge: by confining the learning and wisdom of a generation to one lifetime.

> The "generation gap" is an important social tool for any repressive society. If the younger members of a community view the older members as contemptible or suspect or excess, they will never be able to join hands and examine the living memories of the community, nor ask the all

important question, "Why?" This gives rise to a historical amnesia that keeps us working to invent the wheel every time we have to go to the store for bread. (1984: 117)

Intergenerational allegiances improve the lives of young and old participants. In an interdependent system, friendships and allegiances would no longer be confined within generations, allowing for intergenerational dialogue and a routine engagement with old age and death. As Renee Rose Shield explains, "If friendships outside the family were evenly distributed throughout the age scale, young people would face loss through death as much as old people do. As it is, the old have become a buffer zone between society and death" (1988: 191). That buffer zone is also a buffer between meaningful contact and the rewards of connection. Breaking down that buffer zone can open up new exchanges that can reposition care as an opportunity rather than an obligation. And to do so, we can build on relevant cultural experiences: first, some individuals and families already practice interdependency, and second, attitudes toward dependency at the beginning of life can be expanded to address the spectrum of ability and disability across the life course.

Certainly, interdependency may sound a little idealistic or even unrealistic compared to the more atomized, individualistic approach we currently live with, but interdependency is an experience that some individuals have already had in some pockets and corners, often out of necessity. Interdependency is a requirement for surviving in oppressive conditions. Many minority communities have stronger filial networks that help sustain all generations. These networks provide what social scientists call "parallel services," which are alternatives to or replacements for governmental or private services. Parallel services are necessitated by the expense of traditional services and the history of racism and exclusion in such institutions (Allott and Robb 1998). Pursuing a life characterized by independence is also a function of class privilege. Poor people of all races have to rely on reciprocity, favors, and sharing of resources in order to survive.

One practice that accompanies upward mobility in the United States is to become increasingly distant and atomized as individuals or family units. As a result, interdependency is not entirely unheard of but rather has become increasingly rare among middle- and upper-class families, particularly white families. At Winthrop House, a spirit of being together in the shadow of old age enlivens the community. The prospect of death is real, but it does not dampen the spirit of the place. Recognition and respect are important because they cross class lines. Residents and staff from very different social-class backgrounds embrace their commonalities.

Other advocates and I hope that experiences like those at Winthrop House will provide the seeds for a broader system of interdependency. In an interdependency model, community is sustained through need—not just opportunity—and, as Stephen Kiernan explains, "allowing yourself to be cared for and being a willing recipient of care" becomes a vehicle for contributing to community because such exchanges build up social capital, developing communal ties (2006: 62). At Winthrop House, today's care providers view themselves as future care recipients. They explicitly talk about paying into a cycle of care that will return to them directly as care recipients or to their loved ones. Nurse Beth Jackman makes this cycle of care explicit. Asked about the rewards of her work, she explained, "You want to make sure there's other people that care about that same thing. So they're there to take care of your grandparents for you."

Interdependency does not alleviate inequalities—many of the workers at Winthrop House, especially low-level workers, struggle to survive on the meager wages they receive for providing care that residents rave about. Both residents and workers expressed concern that if the costs of long-term care rise at Winthrop House, or the guidelines for Medicaid change, current workers may never have the chance to become future residents. Yet the frequency with which staff members refer to "when it's my time to move here" indicates that they see themselves engaged in a cycle of care. In fact, Winthrop House president William King is already a resident. And care supervisors Ron Peattie, Clark Daily, and Michael Wood all plan to move to Winthrop House as residents in the years to come.

One kind of likeness—shared racial identity—may be part of the social glue at Winthrop House. Although residents express a desire for the community to become more racially diverse and the community has slowly become so over time, one disquieting possibility is that the monoraciality of Winthrop House actually makes it easier to recognize commonalities than if the residents and the staff represented more diverse racial, ethnic, and cultural backgrounds. Recognition requires one to overlook a whole host of differences that might be divisive outside the walls of Winthrop House, and given the extreme dominance of white people in this social space, it is possible that mutual recognition may be more difficult to sustain in the racially diverse environments that characterize most of the United States and therefore most elder care facilities.

The Imperative for Change

I am arguing for a new practice of interdependency because the way we are handling the longevity dividend right now is not working. In 1982, psychologist Orville Brim and colleagues identified dying as an emergent social problem. They described how the technological innovations of that decade were occurring without clear and effective guidelines about when and how to use them. They argued that if we did not develop such guidelines, "we [would] be ill prepared to meet the more massive accumulative problems that the technology will create tomorrow" (1982: 214). This prescience has grown into a truism in the twenty-first century, when—even more than thirty years after this warning—the American approach to care in old age has not caught up socially and ethically to the conditions made possible by scientific, demographic, and technological change. The warning Brim and colleagues offered in the 1980s has become an imperative in the second decade of the twenty-first century.

As the population of the United States ages, the demographic profile of the citizenry shifts, and the longevity divide continues, several forces are coming to a head that may inspire a reworking of the current approach to old age. I categorize these forces as the economic imperative and the ethical imperative. Economically, the systems we have in place to manage the issues faced by the aging are unsustainable. Scholars agree: "The fundamental problem is that 1 percent of the population accounts for 35 percent of health care spending, [so] the big question is not how we pay for health care, but what are we buying" (Egan 2012). More than in any other country in the world, individuals and the U.S. government pay too much for medical care in the final days of life. Currently, the United States spends more than comparative countries on end-of-life care because most countries put limits on the kinds of procedures and interventions elders undergo by capping social spending. In the United States, one-third of Medicare spending goes to the final year of life, and one-third of that total goes to the final *month* of life (Jacoby 2012). The current debate over how to revamp the medical system in the United States reveals an underlying recognition that the current system is too expensive and inefficient to continue. Medical care for the elderly is at the center of such debates. Experts agree that even if the current act referred to in the popular press as "Obamacare" does not stand, a major revision is needed so that health care costs do not sink the rest of the American economy.

Without a major overhaul, as more Americans live longer lives and accumulate multiple conditions and chronic diseases, the system is likely to implode because of the unavailability of funds for the enormous medical bills that can accrue in the very end of life.

> With a rapidly growing elderly population, with an ever larger share of lives ending gradually, with such a staggering portion of health-care dollars spent on the last months and weeks of life, and with 83 percent of the people who die today covered by Medicare, this equation is fiscally insupportable. (Kiernan 2006: 251)

One likely change is that the United States will look to palliative care to alter the approach to chronic and fatal conditions while cutting costs. A palliative approach to treatment emphasizes doing everything possible to make the patient comfortable, refocusing energy from cure to care and quality. Palliative care is also associated with much lower costs than elaborate medical interventions meant to fight death rather than usher it in.

The second imperative that I describe as ethical is that the current status quo is not only economically unsustainable but also simultaneously unsatisfying. Stephen Kiernan captures the contradictions inherent in the current system.

> Massive spending on end-of-life care would be acceptable if patients were clamoring for ever-more treatments and ever-greater interventions. Instead, they and their families consistently say they want *less* heroics and more pain con-

trol, *less* technology and more compassion. The money is all but being wasted. Ironically, care for the dying is one of those instances in medicine in which *spending more does not result in higher quality.* Dr. Johan Wennberg's studies found no correlation between higher spending and reduced mortality or better end-of-life care. But that data only confirms what most people know intuitively. (2006: 154; italics added)

The heroic lifesaving measures that the medical system can offer are often intrusive and futile in old age. Heroic medical measures not only are costly but also can prevent the more peaceful, quiet conditions many people imagine or hope for in their final days and hours. Interventions may prolong life for a very short amount of time or may require a permanent move to the hospital—a less desirable location for dying than home or a continuing care retirement community (CCRC) that the patient now calls home. Hospitals operate on an emergency model, making intentional leave-taking difficult. It is time for expensive deaths that are traumatic for care recipients to be replaced by a new norm.

The ethical imperative for change arises from the frequency with which people are suffering through the end of their own longevity dividend. One measure of this discontent is how many individuals have begun to put plans in place that limit the scope of medical intervention in certain situations. Living wills, medical power of attorney, do not resuscitate orders (DNRs), wills, and "Five Wishes" are all being used to specify one's goals, desires, and preferences about one's own life and death. Five Wishes is a small packet produced by an organization called Aging with Dignity that walks the author through some scenarios that might occur at the end of life. The cost of Five Wishes is only five dollars, and the form is recognized as a valid health care directive in forty-two states. The increased use of advance directives and hospice speaks to a growing interest in quality of life. For now, these attempts to limit and control the end-of-life process are piecemeal—there is no nationwide system for planning for the end of life. However, what such measures do reveal is that people are concerned about the quality of their lives, interested in controlling their own end, and reluctant to undergo excessive treatments in the later stages of life. These individualized approaches reflect the sentiment surrounding a system that is unsatisfying and too often cruel.

Betting on the Long Tail: Obstacles to Achieving Interdependency

Although the current system for elder care is unsatisfying and unsustainable, viable alternatives have yet to be articulated. In fact, while critics have cautioned the American public and policy makers for years that the United States is unprepared to face global aging, no broad alteration to the current system has been explored. As Mary Pipher explains, although there is some recognition that the current system is broken, the United States has not moved on to building a replacement: "Right now we don't even know how to talk about our problems. We have no language for nurturing interdependency. The traditional ways of caring for our parents don't work, and new ways haven't been invented" (1999: 17). The United States varies from comparative nation-states in this regard because many countries, such as Japan and Canada, have been developing national plans for grappling with global aging for several decades (Act on Social Welfare Service for Elderly 2009; SSCA 2009). By contrast, in the United States, Medicare and Medicaid spending has continued to balloon alongside the uneven development of for-profit and nonprofit institutional "solutions" to elder care.

This lack of a vision for the later years of life is reinforced by a singular focus in medical care on living longer—another day, another week—with very little attention to the how and the why of living longer. Since "fighting death" is the normative model in emergency medicine, facilitating alternative approaches to the end of life requires attention and even vigilance (Kaufman 2005). Dr. Atul Gawande writes about his internal struggle to adhere to individual wishes to extend life regardless of quality. The current medical system, as he explains, is set up to encourage patients and their families to focus on the long shot, or the "long tail," of possible survival with any given terminal illness rather than to focus on how to live for the time remaining.

> There is almost always a long tail of possibility, however thin. What's wrong with looking for it? Nothing, it seems to me, unless it means we have failed to prepare for the outcome that's vastly more probable. The trouble is that we've built our medical system and culture around the long tail. We've created a multitrillion-dollar edifice for dispensing the medical equivalent of lottery tickets—and have only the rudiments of a system to prepare patients for the near-certainty that those tickets will not win. Hope is not a plan, but hope is our plan. (2010: 45)

Doctors, nurses, patients, and family members echo Gawande's observations as they speak out about the undesirable outcomes that often arise when the focus is on prolonging the *length* of the final years rather than expanding the quality. Despite these critiques, the system continues to treat death as a technical failure, as if it were somehow avoidable (Brim et al. 1982: 211). The value Americans place on doing and taking action, combined with an interest in exerting control over nature, situates death as a failure rather than as an unavoidable reality. This perspective too often shapes public discussions of aging and policy. In recent years, the most famous instance of this tendency was how discussions about what Medicare and Medicaid should pay for in the final stages of life led to hyperbolic reports of "death panels."

In 2009, the Obama administration's proposed Health Care Reform Act included a provision in Section 1233 that physicians could be paid to provide voluntary counseling to Medicare patients about end-of-care planning tools, such as living wills, advance directives, and medical power of attorney. Former Republican governor Sarah Palin politicized this minor section of the proposed bill by saying in a speech in August 2009 that the proposed legislation would set up "death panels" that would target elders and individuals with disabilities—such as her child with Down syndrome—to decide who should live and for how long. While Palin's comments were clearly a wide divergence from the truth, she tapped into major fears about decision making at the end of life. Note that the proposed legislation at no time suggested limiting the number of heroic and costly measures provided in the final months of life. Instead, all the proposed legislation suggested was that doctors could be paid to *counsel* elderly patients about their choices and options. The debate became so heated and hyperbolic that the measure had to be struck from the legislation in order to get the act passed. This rare foray into a nationwide discussion about the end of life revealed some true obstacles to reform: many Americans are afraid to plan, and a vocal minority even resent the idea that doctors could advise patients about the end of life. Unfortunately, given these two convictions, for many Americans the only remaining available plan is to ignore the certainty of death until it arrives.

The death panels incident also demonstrated the obstacles to systemic change within the health care and long-term care industries. As hospice chaplain Kerry Egan explained on CNN, addressing the exorbitant costs associated with the last two years of Americans' lives is virtually unspeakable politically.

> President Obama has talked about squeezing billions of waste, fraud and abuse from Medicare. But he has yet to admit the obvious: those savings can only come from changing the way the system treats dying people. About 67 billion—nearly a third of the money spent by Medicare—goes to patients in the last two years of life. The need to spend less money at the end of life "is the elephant in the room," Evan Thomas wrote in "The Case for Killing Granny," the cover story in last week's *Newsweek*. Everyone sees it but no one wants to talk about it. (2012: 2)

In exchange for not having a different national conversation about medical care, aging, quality of life, and death, the United States pays an extraordinary national bill for medical interventions (particularly in the last year of life) that are often unsuccessful and unsatisfying.

Currently, needs in old age divide us rather than unite us. This is because there are deep philosophical differences about human rights and social goods and because social inequality constrains the full possibilities of the longevity dividend. Although Medicare and Medicaid financially support many elders, the decisions, locations, and systems for providing care must be individually accessed and arranged. As a result, the options available to individual families vary considerably according to the financial resources of the family, the social networks and resources of the family, and the social location of the elder in terms of race, gender, class, and region. Medicare and Medicaid recipients have different options than private pay families and elders. Racial minorities have fewer options than majority elders. Small towns and rural areas offer different options than do cities. Different parts of the country specialize in different forms of care. Some cities offer faith-specific care or specialize according to residents' occupations or sexual orientation. By contrast, elders who wish to live out their days in small towns have few if any options. Options for providing in-home care are also often linked to class and location.

The refusal of the nation-state to offer systemic support for elders is supported by societal attitudes that increasingly situate elders as drains on the system. Meredith Minkler and Thomas Cole (1999) argue that attitudes toward elderly citizens became increasingly negative in the second half of the twentieth century. Rather than being viewed as powerful or venerable citizens in the United States, elders are "blamed" in political debates for having needs and are situated as a greedy collective that steals resources from younger generations (Browne 1998). Debates about what elders deserve continue unabated and are likely to heat up as the proportion of old to young dramatically shifts in the coming twenty years. Unless we identify and embrace a plan that alters the perception of a zero-sum game between elders and other beneficiaries of attention, time, care, and fiscal support, the differences between age groups are likely to become sites of conflict (Callahan 1987). Most demographers anticipate that in the United States the elder boom will peak around 2030. Other national dilemmas threaten to add fuel to this potential intergenerational battle: high unemployment among young Americans, greater wealth concentrated among the baby boomers as compared to younger generations, and the potential insolvency of Social Security, Medicaid, and Medicare. In the meantime, the social support structure for our longer lives remains spotty to insufficient.

What would it be like if we, as a nation, found a way around the often futile expenditures toward a different approach to the final years of life? What would it take to foster an approach that views death as natural and normal, not something to be fought against? An interdependent practice would recognize the spectrum of ability and disability that characterizes our own lives and would situate the time preceding death as one step along that continuum. To develop an alternative viewpoint like this, we must rethink our attitudes toward dependency.

The Myth of Independence

Right now, elder care is viewed as a private responsibility best attended to by family members. Situating elder care as a private responsibility rather than a collective one is stressful for families while also being consistent with dearly held American ideals such as self-reliance and individualism. The ideal of independence often drives beliefs and behaviors in the United States, both for better and for worse. The United States declared independence at its founding, teenagers declare independence to announce their adulthood, and childhood is marked by a series of stages of increasing independence. By contrast, we have few rituals to mark and support the other kinds of changes—moves toward greater dependency.

During our lives we actually do not move into independence and stay there, but rather our needs and abilities vary consistently over time. Self-reliance is largely a myth, even at middle age. Most of us are dependent on older and younger family members, friends, neighbors, coworkers, mentors, and service providers to keep our daily lives stable and flowing smoothly. Personal changes that require increased dependency include chronic conditions, times of illness, recovery after surgery, and pregnancy. Needs become even more pronounced in the later years of life when our bodies and minds impose new limits on pure independence. In short, while courage, perseverance, and a commitment to doing as much as one can may help elders feel strong and capable, trying to maintain absolute independence is simply a losing battle during the eighth, ninth, and tenth decades of life.

Dependency is often treated as avoidable rather than routine, ordinary, and predictable (Baltes 1996: 11). Too frequently, dependency in adults is not recognized as a simple expression of need or of having reached a personal limit, but rather it is attributed to a personal lack or failure. As Margaret Baltes points out, "This alignment has catastrophic consequences, since it justified taking over the lives of people thus deemed incompetent and denying them freedom, choice, and privacy" (1996: 11). When dependency is viewed as a "problem" rather than a predictable reality, it sets up a crisis response to what is a common life experience: needing help. Treating dependency as an individual failure prevents the gathering of resources and insights to build security nets that might be available to all. And when that help is viewed as the sole responsibility of families to provide or arrange, it obscures the collective challenges of living and aging in a society in which old age is more common than youth.

Framing dependency as failure also discourages elders from acknowledging their own needs for assistance and asking for help. As Mary Pipher explains, elders often pass judgment on their own changing needs. "They don't want to be a burden, the greatest of American crimes. [Elders] often feel ashamed of what is a natural stage of the life cycle. . . . If we view life as a time line, we realize that all of us are sometimes more and sometimes less dependent on others" (1999: 51). As the disability rights movement has accurately pointed out, the dual assumptions that ability and independence are normal and natural set up a situation in which need and interdependency take on a negative hue.

The negative evaluation of dependency also promotes policies that situate the services and support needed to address dependency as properly provided by the dependent adults and their family, not by a wider support network. In fact, culturally in the United States, our fear of death and our distrust of dependency combine to work against planning and vision for elder care. In place of planning, we cling to the hope that somehow the dependencies that are predictable in adulthood will be sidestepped and avoided through good health and good luck. Like the gambling on the "long tail" survival of terminally ill patients that Dr. Gawande pointed out, we bet on the unlikely event that we will remain entirely independent until the moment of our death. Likewise, we shape policies that sustain the myth of independence rather than create a cultural context that could support and sustain interdependency and the exchange of care over time.

In addition to changing attitudes toward dependency, inventing new ways of caring for elders and nurturing interdependency will require overcoming the social and even spatial distance between generations. As Bonnie Cashin Farmer explains, one of the costs of segregating elders from younger generations is that young people begin to "see older people as different from themselves; thus they subtly cease to identify with older individuals as human beings" (1996: 120). Mutual recognition is a crucial foundation for interdependency, and spatial segregation discourages such recognition. Laura Katz Olson points out that generational segregation practically ensures that we will not recognize one another. Writing about elders, she ponders, "Perhaps hiding them away spares us 'a confrontation with our own future'" (2003: 242). Holding elders' experiences at bay supports a strategy of denial rather than compassionate action. We sustain the (unlikely) hope that we will never be the recipient of assistance. If we bank on that long shot, we fail to do the work it takes to build and sustain a system of support from which each of us can draw at the time we need it.

The sequestering of the old also allows us to maintain the fallacy of being whole, complete, sanitized, hygienic, and bounded, but this kind of boundedness is purely illusion. As Daniel Callahan explains so beautifully, "To be mortal is to live a life that will be marked by illness, injury, aging, decline, and death. . . . Human beings will and must be a burden on one another; the flight from dependency is a flight from humanity" (1993: 123–127). We temporarily maintain a sense of independence only to fail at it later. And one of the costs of trying to sustain this farce is the segregation of old age and the ignorance we willfully maintain about the dilemmas and dependencies we are headed toward in our final days. Shifting attitudes toward dependency will take some work, but the road to interdependency includes well-traveled territory. To achieve an outlook consistent with interdependent practice, we need only extend the compassion we feel toward potential and needs of the young to potential and needs of the old.

Birth and Death

Like birth, dying is one of life's most pivotal experiences. It demands attention to the physical body and the spiritual, psychological, and social self. Death, like labor, demands skill, courage, and knowledge. We are born, and we die. We do a better job helping one another enter life than helping one another exit life. What if we treat dying not like an untouchable or profane time of life but instead like a sacred or noble passage that is deeply human, that connects us in its commonness?

Many of the workers I interviewed bemoaned the lack of rituals to sustain the changes at the end of life as compared with those that prepare the ground for the arrival of a new person. Chaplain Phyllis Star says, "There's a tremendous preparation for people when they're born, and then after that, it diminishes as you go along. And so at the end, there is no celebration." Even before a baby is born, a community gathers and prepares a space of support. Baby showers, birthing classes, advice from parents, and offers of assistance all mark the upcoming arrival. The arrival of an entirely dependent being is met with offers of assistance, a pooling of resources, and new allegiances of support. Stephen Kiernan contrasts the wealth of resources surrounding a child with the lack of resources surrounding many elders.

> Some of society's most embracing actions come in the community that forms around a new person. The entrance to life could not be more different from the exit. People spend their final days in hospitals or nursing homes, often with little more companionship than a TV. As they become sicker, friends back away and doctors abandon them. Too often life's end is also its loneliest phase. (2006: 159)

Those who labor at the end of life see many parallels between their work and the work of ushering in a new life. Hospice nurse Eva Crowley likens her work to being a midwife. "It's like being a midwife, with birthing, you know: everyone's going to die, we're all going to die. It's kind of a special time. As humans, we're all going to be there." Sandra Blossom, a family caregiver who helped her mother-in-law until she was too ill to be at home and then took care of her with the help of CCRC and hospice staff, compared her experience to being a witness to and participant in a birth.

> The one thing about that whole process was that it really frames death as a part of life. It really frames it as a natural, very sad event, but something that you can participate in or be involved with or, you know, somehow partake in

at a very . . . I don't want to say spiritual level because I'm not very religious, but at a humanity level. It's so human—it was very difficult to go through, but it was also very rewarding in that it's almost like how people feel when you give birth. Like it's a privilege and an honor to watch a life come into the world, and I almost felt the same way—not that I wanted her to die. Her being sick was awful, but those last hours, you know, I kind of felt the same way, with a lot more sadness than joy like the birth of a baby—that's very joyful and this is more sad, but it's almost the same feeling for me.

Elder care providers can again provide a model for how to move forward and honor the end of life as a time not to be mourned but to be acknowledged, embraced, and even celebrated.

To start rethinking dependency and reduce the divides between generations, we need to view old age with the same recognition and tenderness that we ordinarily extend to infancy. The labor of raising infants is visible and supported. Sometimes it even reduces the social space between people: friends, neighbors, and coworkers may help the parents-to-be before and just after the birth of the child by visiting, contributing food or gifts, and helping to care for the new infant. At the end of life, elders exhibit parallels to infancy: in the latest part of life they may sleep a lot, speak less frequently, need help walking, require assistance with eating and drinking, and even need help in getting to places and seeing and doing the things they enjoy. Like infants, elders increasingly need the help of others to maintain their bodies: elders' skin becomes even more delicate, and they may need help going to the bathroom, turning in bed, or bathing. Like the early part of life, the late part of life may require special equipment, including walkers, diapers, specialized beds, or pureed foods. And yet, too often, we rail against these needs. The needs at the start of life are often perceived as cute, quaint, and even beautiful. We are enchanted with need at the beginning of life, yet we mourn similar needs in old age. Clearly, the ascent into personhood from infancy is part of the human project. People talk about birth and new personhood as miraculous and marvelous. Those who usher others toward death often have the same feeling: that they are engaged in meaningful work that is deeply human. What might it look like to approach death with a sense of awe and humility rather than dread? Here again, the elders at Winthrop House offer some insights into the possibility of clearly anticipating life's final chapter.

A Well-Planned Final Chapter

My time at Winthrop House has inspired me to imagine much larger spaces where talk about aging and death is frank and unromantic. Studying the longevity dividend has led me to believe that in the United States (and, similarly, in other advanced, industrialized countries) we are entering a stage of history that is going to require new types of courage and innovation. And as I talk to people who are actively engaged in the frontiers of old age, I think we will discover new capacities and gifts along the way. One example of these new opportunities is that at Winthrop House, the vast majority of residents have planned their own death. In the United States, the percentage of elders with advance directives is less than 30 percent, but at Winthrop House, a remarkable sixty-nine of the seventy people I surveyed had put plans in place for some or *all* of the dying process (PBS *Frontline* 2010). Residents had named legal decision makers, talked through possible scenarios with the person to whom they had granted medical power of attorney, secured commitments from family members, written obituaries, paid for burials, and made arrangements for their belongings and money to be given away, and even for their bodies to be donated. One resident said, "I have made plans and keep revising and updating them. Are they adequate? That will be up to my survivors to decide!" Another resident wrote in one sentence about the dread of a too-long dying and the measures she had put in place: "My plan (hope) is to go quickly, to be the subject of no funeral or 'celebration of life,' and to have my carcass delivered to the (local) medical school for its use in instruction." Their planning is frank and sometimes even funny. For example, one resident said she had arranged for her body to be donated to a local university. "I hope they take well-used parts!" she said. Their stated reasons for such careful plans were that they do not want to burden children or other relatives with decisions about what to do after their death, but it is clear that their planning has also freed them up. One resident says, "One should never leave loose ends when it comes to dying." Their plans reflect a sober engagement with death that remains a rarity in most of American culture.

Residents' planning reveals an intentional engagement with death and an extension of the power and control that these people apply in their daily life. Resident Aida Dorenfield explains how she and her husband have planned at length and talked with their children in detail. She says that because her own father had a living will, she was able to make decisions that limited the life-prolonging procedures that he dreaded.

> [I could decide *not* to] do a hip replacement even though there was a surgeon very willing to operate on a ninety-year-old man who had no idea who he was or where he was and would never be able to do the physical therapy required to walk again. We have read the statistics of how much of our health care dollars go to the last few months of life in th[is] country, and we hope we aren't going to add

to the problem. We would rather have better schools, better infrastructure, and a country not burdened with huge debt to leave to our children.

The decision to dictate and control end-of-life decisions before the time arrives is presented as an act of respect toward younger relatives and, in the case of Aida, a gift to an entire generation: she would rather have funds directed toward building durable collective services than add a few days or weeks to her or her husband's life.

Like their frank talk about daily life, the nearly universal preparedness of Winthrop House residents is revealing. Such planning requires foresight about and insight into what can happen in the absence of well-laid plans. It also requires trusting those who are left in charge of one's belongings and body to follow through when the person can no longer make decisions. Several residents explained their decisions in terms of having learned from the example (both good and bad) of friends and neighbors. They also made clear that their plans were dependent on trusting the staff of Winthrop House to follow the directions they have put in place. Resident Mary Beth Kleinschmidt explains how her plans rely on her trust of both her children and the workers at Winthrop House.

> I wonder if my [husband and I] will be able to remain in our home to the end or if we will need to take advantage of increasing levels of care. I realize our situation could change quickly, and I also realize that much depends on my ability to make it possible for Thomas to remain at home. We know that Winthrop House will help us with these decisions, as will our children.

This group of elders will not be caught off guard by death—they want a say, even after life has left their bodies. They talk about it as a gift to younger relatives, and what a gift it is! Their planning is also a way of settling their own affairs so that the specter of death holds less power. Once the plans are laid, the prospect of death takes less energy, leaving more energy and time to live out the days and years before death arrives. Describing parts of Winthrop House, Mary Beth's husband, Thomas Kleinschmidt, even said, "I remember thinking during the dedication of the new care center that I would probably die in that building." The couple's approach to the inevitable end of their lives includes no self-delusion and little fanfare. Their planning is not a form of submission; instead, it represents intentional planning based on trust in their relatives and the staff at Winthrop House.

Imagining an Interdependent Future

Some mornings I wake up very early with my son, Erik. In those quiet predawn hours, I imagine that I can hear the human world awakening: a truck driver trudges out to his truck amid the hissing of the engine; a farmer wakes before the roosters to spread feed for her chickens and goats; a coffee shop worker switches on the lights, grinds the beans, brews the coffee; parents like me rock babies or stroke fevered foreheads; and all the people—children, spouses, home care workers, and elder care workers—rise to care for the old and ailing. Chaplains sit with those who may not live until dawn. Nurse's aides raise beds, pick out clothes, slide on shoes, offer water and coffee, and inquire, "How did you sleep, Gloria? Was it a good night?" I think about the rustling of bodies, old and young, that are being helped lovingly and willfully to rest comfortably as the sun rises.

We are already reliant on one another to make it through the day to face the dawn. Developing interdependent practice will require us to revalue and recenter our connections with one another to form an intentional practice of interdependency. The potential rewards of embracing interdependency are many. Like the experts who reap the rewards of helping others die in ways that honor their preferences and histories, we all have an opportunity to affect the aging and dying processes of our friends, our family, and ourselves. As we take on the labor of aging and dying as important work—work that parallels birth in its significance—we discover new capacities within ourselves, and new possibilities at the end of life. Experts talk about finding the freedom to face death, the maturity to accompany others as they die, the power to influence how someone feels about approaching death, and the satisfaction of having used one's skills in the service of something so important. Janet Conroy felt that she had made an important contribution when she cared for her mother. When asked what advice she would give to another family caregiver whose loved one had just received a terminal diagnosis, she said, "I would tell [the caregiver] that they give you support in ways you never imagined. It turns what could be a really frightening experience, if you're open to it, to what's absolutely one of life's amazing experiences." Like the experts in CCRCs and hospices who help others die every day, Janet says that helping her mother die was an amazing experience with the advantage of hindsight. For those of us who have yet to have the experience, we must trust and take a leap of hope that death for us can also be amazing. Embracing interdependency also allows us to face the certainty of our own and our loved ones' death with courage and purpose rather than avoidance and fear.

Transforming our culture into one grounded in interdependent practice will begin to address the social changes wrought by a rapidly aging culture. It will allow people who are already older to draw on broader and deeper reserves of help. Interdependency is not a plan that simply seeks to support and sustain only individuals who have unmet needs for assistance in the later years of life, but rather a plan that will assist all participants. Elders will be expected and encouraged to contribute to networks of mutual recognition and support. In an interdependent practice, elders will benefit from the attention and support of a broader group, and elders will be expected to share their skills: making music, sewing clothes, maintaining gardens, recounting history, and providing food. In an interdependent approach, elder care facilities will house day care centers and pet adoption programs. Neighborhoods will receive incentives for including wheelchair-accessible housing, and schools will include education about the life course and contact with local elders.

Interdependency relies on a shift from looking at care needs as an obligation to viewing them as an opportunity: a chance to contribute to the community store of sustenance and goodwill. Within an interdependency model, caring for elders becomes an honor and an opportunity, not a burden (Pipher 1999: 52). As Mary Pipher explains, taking care of elders provides younger generations with an opportunity to "repay our parents for the love they gave us, and it is our last chance to become grownups. We help them to help ourselves" (1999: 52). Dependency in old age gives adult children the chance to care for their parents as their parents did for them, and it gives friends and family the opportunity to show love and concern through thoughtful acts, presence, and support. Receiving care from others at the end of life also gives the dying person an opportunity to teach. During the dying process, we learn from elders about courage, dealing with pain, and what really matters after a life has been lived.

The idea that the dying give us something reminds me of a story told by a family care provider named Sandra Blossom. Sandra cared for her mother-in-law, Mary Richter, on what turned out to be the last day of her life. When Mary's nurse asked Sandra if she would like to help wash her mother-in-law, together the two women lifted Mary's pained body. They took sponges and wet her head, arms, and feet. They changed her bedding and gave her a fresh nightgown. Mary moaned at times, and Sandra was unsure if they should continue, but the nurse assured her that this sort of loving touch was a way to communicate when words had long passed. After an hour or so, Sandra and the nurse settled Mary back into a clean bed, and later that night she died. Sandra said with great pride and tears in her voice, "I did that. I washed her for the last time. I was able to give her something on her last day." Sandra and Mary's story speaks to the awe-inspiring effects of laboring at the end of life. In Sandra's case, she was invited by a nurse to roll up her sleeves and take responsibility for her mother-in-law's dying body. The result was that she felt proud that she had found the strength not to help Mary die, but rather to help her as she was dying: to get her ready to go on her final day.

Sandra's story is also an example of how professionals and family providers can join forces to accompany someone to death. As ethicist Daniel Callahan explains, recognizing one another's needs and capacities is essential, since our futures is likely to include care from both familiar and less familiar others.

> Because of our increasingly extended old age, there is a good chance that many of us will die in the company of strangers, our spouses and friends dead before us, and perhaps even our children. We would do well to hope those strangers will have a sensitivity to death, that they will know how to talk with and to comfort us, and that they will see in our dying their own eventual fate and thus our common lot. (1993: 227–228)

Our lack of preparation for the end of life must be overcome and systematically addressed. The gap between our current system and an interdependent practice is not that wide; we already have the resources we need to move to the new system. The latent connections between us simply need to be enlivened and activated so that when the changes associated with aging and dying kick in, we can witness, support, and accompany as we do with the journey *into* life. We could have community elder care classes, offer seminars on adapting to old age, and increase the incentives for professionals to pursue elder care and gerontology. In fact, honoring the labor of dying and accompanying one another in that process are in many ways less complicated and certainly less costly than endless medical interventions.

Like other important labors in life, accompanying other persons through the threshold of elongated dying can provide the gratification of doing a hard task well, the value of using one's skills to help another person be comfortable, and the pleasure of offering support and having that support received with gratitude. For those who are the recipients of care in communities that are truly interdependent, there is the additional satisfaction of knowing that this exchange, what Stephen Kiernan calls the "ultimate intimacy," was also part of a network of exchanges to which they once did or will contribute as well, each to his or her own power and abilities. As the balance between old age and youth shifts, there will be more scenes of the type Sandra Blossom describes and fewer scenes of crying babies in delivery rooms. Last baths will be more common than first baths. The longevity dividend is our communal inheritance; how we approach it—reluctantly or willfully—is still to be determined. The time to prepare is now.

Afterword

I wrote this book in part to prepare myself to take care of my dad later in his life. By age fifty, my dad had been in and out of the hospital with multiple chronic conditions exacerbated by drinking and obesity. Dad loved sports and continued to play tennis, basketball, or golf almost every day despite his multiple health challenges, so some of his visits to the doctor were to replace or repair strained "parts" like torn ligaments and broken bones. When he was fifty-eight years old, my dad went into a coma after a particularly difficult bout of pneumonia. He stayed in the coma for sixteen days. My sister and I struggled to know what to do. He had no medical power of attorney, no living will, and no do not resuscitate (DNR) order. However, we knew enough to realize he would not want to be kept in a hospital for the rest of his days. Despite my dad's poor health before that particular hospital visit, little prepared us for moving from living with illness to moving toward death. Our sixteen days in that threshold revealed how ill prepared we were to care for him—or later, to care for our mom or each other when the time came.

My dad came back from the threshold that time. In fact, although he never came back to 100 percent after that bleak month of February 2004, he lived long enough to retire to Florida, to meet one of his grandsons, and to play many more tennis matches. Having had that close call, Dad and I started making more deliberate plans about what he wanted: he gave me medical power of attorney, he told me where his belongings were and what he wanted for his cremation, and we talked about his fears. If my sister and I ended up at his bedside in a hospital again, we would be ready this time.

Then one November night in 2011, Dad fell in his bathroom and died—probably of a stroke or heart attack, we do not know for sure. So I never needed to make the difficult decisions that he and I both feared. My sister and I never returned to a bedside like the one we kept watch at in 2004.

Dad died the way old men used to die: suddenly. I remain somewhat grateful for the suddenness of his death. By the time my dad retired to Florida in the early 2000s, he was on more than twenty drugs per day and experiencing all the challenges associated with drug interactions. My dad was also haunted by the fear of becoming dependent on me or my sister. His death saved him from ever having to move to a nursing home or continuing care retirement community or to live with me and my family as he feared he would someday need to. He did not experience a slow decline that emptied the bank accounts he had worked to fill on a meager teacher's salary. Many of his fears were waylaid. I can comfort myself by thinking that my dad had the quick end that he said he would prefer.

And yet, my dad missed out on the longevity dividend. Born in 1946, he did not get the extra decades that so many of his contemporaries are now enjoying. And despite the health challenges that would have continued to accelerate and plague him had he lived longer, he also missed out on so much that those extra days—even years—might have provided: the opportunity to celebrate the first birthday of a grandchild, to see another president inaugurated, to witness another spring, to watch the sun go down over the ocean, to talk about a movie or a book that he loved, to tell a story, or to call his daughter on a Sunday morning. It seems to me that whatever sudden deaths save us from, more days on this planet, more days spent together would be the real gift. Our challenge now is to gather all of our insights and ingenuity, our resources, and our compassion and figure out how to make the labor at the end of life a rewarding experience, not one to be feared.

Glossary

ADLs (activities of daily living): Activities including eating, bathing, grooming, dressing, walking, toileting, and getting in and out of bed or on and off chairs.

Advance directive: A legal document making provisions for decision making if an individual becomes incapable of making medical decisions for himself or herself. Advance directives include assigning a medical power of attorney, a will, or a Five Wishes document.

Aging in place: An industry term describing the goal of allowing elders to stay in one place, with services remaining available to them as their needs vary over time. The "in place" may be a long-term private home or part of a long-term care facility. This approach is a new standard in elder care. In previous eras, elders had to go wherever the services they needed were provided. In this model, the service providers go wherever the elder person resides.

Alzheimer's disease: A degenerative disease that affects the brain, named after Dr. Alois Alzheimer, a German neurologist who identified what he called "presenile dementia." The cause is still being researched, and treatments can slow but do not reverse the effects of the illness. Those suffering from the disease progress from some short-term memory loss and occasional dementia to an almost complete retreat into alternative social worlds. As lives have extended, the Alzheimer's rate has grown dramatically. For example, among those over the age of eighty-five, the frequency rate is now one in two individuals.

Ambiguous dying: The uncertainties characteristic of prolonged dying. As Mercedes Bern-Klug (2004) explains, chronic and degenerative diseases make it difficult to know when a person is transitioning from living with illness to actively dying. Part of the job of end-of-life workers is to help friends, families, and the patients themselves recognize the signs of approaching death, to make the dying process less ambiguous.

Assisted living: A format for elder care developed in the late twentieth century that provides minimal assistance in terms of medical care and/or activities of daily living. Assisted living generally denotes less total care than a nursing home. In a continuing care retirement community, assisted living may be one of the "stages" of care that is offered as a resident's needs change.

Baby boomers: Individuals born in the United States between 1946 and 1965 (Howe and Strauss 1991). The term *baby boomers* refers to this large generation of people born immediately after World War II. Other nations that engaged in the war experienced similar population bumps as young soldiers returned from war and raised families.

Burden of choice: A term I devised to describe the pressure that elders and their friends and caregivers feel as a result of technological and medical advancements. Prolonged dying presents a series of "junctures" requiring decisions about whether or not to pursue medical treatments and/or which treatments to pursue. These choices generate new burdens that did not exist in previous generations, when the therapies and technologies were not yet available and the dying processes were therefore both quicker and more opaque.

CCRC (continuing care retirement community): An age-specific resident living community that offers a range of service provisions from independent living to round-the-clock nursing care. A growing option for elder living, CCRCs usually require that residents pay a move-in fee and a monthly fee to live in the community. An advantage of CCRCs is that residents can access a range of services over time without moving; for couples, both people can live in the same community even if one needs more assistance than the other.

Death experts: My term for workers who have acquired significant occupational knowledge through their experience in caring for the dying. Death experts include the elder care facility workers I interviewed for this book, as well as funeral directors, religious leaders, grief counselors, and the like.

Death novices: People who have limited experience with or knowledge about death. Most of us are death novices.

Demography: The statistical study of human populations. As it relates to aging, demography can help reveal changes in the proportion of elders as compared with other age cohorts, changes in life expectancy, and changes in fertility. The notion of global aging refers to a planet-wide demographic trend—the aging of the human population in most nations.

Dependency ratio: The proportion of individuals actively working in a society that can support those who are not in the labor force. This calculation helps capture the balance between young adults and old adults in a particular society (Baltes 1996).

Dilemmas of the threshold: A concept I developed to encompass the challenges caused by prolonged living and ambiguous dying. Here, I identify the "threshold" as an indeterminate state between actively living and actively dying. The dilemmas of the threshold are all the uncertainties that attach to the longer process of moving from being alive to being dead, including, for example, how to treat the person who may be dying, what medical interventions to pursue, and when to start talking about approaching death.

DNR (do not resuscitate) order: An advance directive that stipulates that if breathing stops, the person does not want to be resuscitated through CPR. DNR orders apply at home, in a hospital, or in a nursing home. Any adult can write a DNR order. But DNR orders are particularly common among elders who are chronically ill, since CPR is not always successful and resumed breathing can be accompanied by brain damage or other limitations to quality of life. Unfortunately, DNR orders are not always honored, since medical professionals do not always inquire about DNR orders prior to resuscitation.

Elongated lives: A term I developed in conjunction with "prolonged dying" to describe the two primary changes in how we live and die now: we live longer and die more slowly than our ancestors.

Emotional labor: A term developed by Arlie Hochschild (1983) to describe the production of feeling states in exchange for a wage. For example, service workers may be required to exhibit specific emotions, such as friendliness, cheerfulness, and excitement, as part of their jobs.

Fertility rate: A statistical prediction of the expected number of children who will be born to a woman of childbearing years. Since the 1960s, widely available over-the- counter birth control and women's movements around the world have greatly reduced the fertility rate. In the United States, the current fertility rate is below "replacement rate" (the rate at which the population is sustained in size). In 2010, the fertility rate was 2.1, as compared with a fertility rate above 3.5 in the 1960s.

Five Wishes: The organization Aging with Dignity developed a document called the Five Wishes, which asks five questions to determine who should make medical decisions if a patient cannot and what the patient's beliefs and values are about medical intervention, death, and postdeath remembrances. Five Wishes costs five dollars and is recognized as a legal advance directive in forty-two states (available at http://www.agingwithdignity.org/five-wishes.php).

Gendered aging: A term that encompasses the multiple differences in aging between the genders. Examples include the fact that women live longer than men in almost every nation, that women constitute the majority of both unpaid and paid caregivers to elders, and that women and men have very different survival rates for different diseases.

Global aging: A phenomenon that the United Nations described in the 1990s as the "silent revolution" of the dramatic aging of many societies (United Nations 2000). Most developed nations now have programs dedicated to the study of global aging (e.g., the U.S. Administration on Aging), which seek to understand and plan for the economic, social, and environmental consequences of the aging of human populations in the twenty-first century.

Hospice: An approach to the care of terminally ill people that emphasizes comfort and quality of life in the time that remains, an open acknowledgment of approaching death, and a rejection of life-prolonging medical techniques. Hospice, which derives from the French word for "host," began as a formal approach to care for dying people developed by Dr. Cicely Saunders in England in the 1960s (Saunders 1990). The approach quickly grew in popularity and spread to nearby nations. Hospice care can be provided in a hospice house or in the home or elder facility where a patient lives. In the United States, a patient must be identified as having less than six months to live to be eligible for hospice care, whereas in other nations hospice is the tail end of a larger system of palliative care (care that focuses on comfort rather than life-prolonging measures). Although many patients and families associate hospice with dying faster, studies show that patients who receive hospice care often live longer. Hospice is philosophically driven, but it has also been found to curb costs of care in the final stages of life.

IADLs (instrumental activities of daily living): Activities that include housekeeping, laundry, and other maintenance chores; shopping; food preparation; managing money; and paying bills.

Illusion of control: The illusion often produced by advances in medical technology that patients and their friends and families have choices about when or how to die and therefore have control over the time or cause of death.

Industrialization: An economic change—one that has major social consequences—in which the organization of human effort primarily follows the rules and tendency of industry. Efficiency becomes the preeminent standard for how to function. Industrialization of a nation is often accompanied by urbanization (the shift of the majority of the population from rural residence to urban residence). In the realm of old age, industrialization is associated with a decrease in familiarity with death—parts of life are increasingly compartmentalized and professionalized so that many individuals live as death novices.

Life expectancy: The number of years that a person is statistically likely to live. Life expectancy has increased dramatically in the past century, as much as thirty years in some countries.

Living will: A legal document specifying that if the prospect of a meaningful recovery is minimal, the individual prefers to be allowed to die rather than be kept alive by artificial means.

Longevity dividend: My term for the extra years of life that many humans can now expect to live. This "dividend" is the result of preventive health care, improved nutrition, and lifesaving medical advances that prolong life and prevent some previously unpreventable deaths. Many humans today can expect to live as much as thirty years longer than their recent ancestors. I contend that whether the longevity dividend is treated as a problem or as an opportunity depends on education and planning.

Neoliberalism: A political philosophy and practice that highly values privatization of previously public goods and services. The rise of neoliberalism is associated with President Ronald Reagan in the United States and Prime Minister Margaret Thatcher in England in the 1980s. Neoliberalism distrusts government to provide goods and services, celebrating instead the efficiency of the marketplace to perform this function. As a result, neoliberalism is associated with deregulation.

Nursing home: A privately owned (profit or nonprofit) organization that provides full-time nursing care for elderly, disabled, or temporarily disabled residents who cannot care for themselves. Often, elder facilities are referred to as nursing homes even if they do not provide full-time nursing care.

Palliative care: Care that seeks to ease the discomfort associated with a disease rather than cure the illness. Palliative care can moderate the intensity of care and offer comfort to patients at any stage of a disease or any stage of life. Hospice is an end-of-life version of palliative care.

Privatization: The change from public control of a service to private ownership and control.

Prolonged dying: A term I developed to describe the gradual and incremental deaths that characterize the experience today in contrast to the sudden deaths that were more common in the past. Prolonged dying and elongated lives are the two most important trends in how we die now.

Rationalization: The process, in connection with industrialization, by which parts of life or life processes are brought under the control of principles of scientific management. Rationalization streamlines human processes by emphasizing efficiency, productivity, downsizing, and predictability. Rationalization also has negative side effects. It has been associated with decreased wages and decreased quality of life for workers.

Replacement rate: The total number of children each female newborn would need to give birth to in order to replace the total population. If no children died before reaching adulthood, that number would be 2.0—one male and one female born to each female. Taking mortality into consideration, replacement rates range between 2 and 4. Because many countries now have a fertility rate that is below the replacement rate, the total global population is expected to decrease in coming years.

Role reversal: For two people, the act of taking on each other's normal or expected roles. In end-of-life care, an example is when a resident, who would normally be expected to receive care and concern from a worker, extends care and concern to a worker instead.

Structural racism: The regular and systemic privileging of the needs and interests of white people over the needs and interests of people of color, including preferential treatment of white people and discrimination against people of color. In terms of aging, structural racism affects the quality of care elders receive, the range and quality of services available, and even life expectancy.

Technological brinkmanship: A set of challenges posed by the availability of new medical technologies. Doctors are trained to offer all available technologies, and patients are uncertain about whether they can or should decline treatments. Once a therapy or intervention is started, it opens the door to additional procedures. Technological brinkmanship seeks to capture the complexities of these dynamics (Callahan 1993).

Threshold: A concept I developed to describe the ambiguous space and time between living and dying that has become a more common experience. The term captures the liminality of the time (sometimes days, sometimes years) during which a person is living with a deadly illness that will eventually terminate his or her life.

Total institution: A concept developed by sociologist Erving Goffman (1961) to describe spaces where similarly situated people live together isolated from the larger culture and lead a formally ordered and managed life. Nursing homes are considered total institutions.

Will: A legal document defining in advance of death how an individual wants his or her assets and personal effects to be distributed.

References

Abel, Emily K., and Margaret K. Nelson, eds. 1990. *Circles of Care: Work and Identity in Women's Lives.* Albany: State University of New York Press.

Ackerman, Diane. 2011. "The Lonely Polar Bear." *New York Times,* June 2, p. SR9.

Act on Social Welfare Service for Elderly. 2009. Updated April 1, 2009. Translated by Liting Cong. Available at http://www.japaneselawtrans lation.go.jp. Accessed May 18, 2011.

"Aging Population in Spain." 2007. Available at http://news-spain.euro residentes.com/2007/03/ageing-population-in-spain.html.

Allott, Margaret, and Martin Robb. 1998. *Understanding Health and Social Care: An Introductory Reader.* London: Sage.

Alzheimer's Association. 2010. Available at www.alz.org.

Anders, George. 1997. *Health against Wealth: HMOs and the Breakdown of Medical Trust.* Boston: Houghton Mifflin.

Angel, Ronald J., and Jacqueline L. Angel. 1997. *Aging and Long-Term Care in Multicultural America.* New York: New York University Press.

Baltes, Margaret M. 1996. *The Many Faces of Dependency in Old Age.* Cambridge: Cambridge University Press.

Beauvoir, Simone de. 1970. *The Coming of Age.* Paris: Editions Gallimard.

Bern-Klug, Mercedes. 2004. "The Ambiguous Dying Syndrome." *Health and Social Work* 29 (1): 55–64.

Bosch, Xavier. 2000. "Spain Faces Massive Decline in Population." *British Medical Journal* 320 (7239): 891.

Botsford, Flora. 2002. "Ageing: Spain's Dilemma." April 9. *BBC News.*

Brabant, Sarah. 2003. "Death in Two Settings: The Acute Care Facility and Hospice." In *Handbook of Death and Dying,* edited by Clifton D. Bryant, 475–484. New York: Sage.

Brim, Orville G., Jr., Howard E. Freeman, Sol Levine, and Norman A. Scotch, eds. 1982. *The Dying Patient.* New York: Russell Sage Foundation.

Brown, Michael. 2004. "Between Neoliberalism and Cultural Conservatism: Spatial Division and Multiplications of Hospice Labor in the United States." *Gender, Place, and Culture* 11 (1): 67–82.

Browne, Colette V. 1998. *Women, Feminism, and Aging.* New York: Springer Publishing.

Byock, Ira. 1997. *Dying Well: Peace and Possibilities at the End of Life.* New York: Riverhead Books.

Callahan, Daniel. 1987. *Setting Limits: Medical Goals in an Aging Society.* New York: Simon and Schuster.

———. 1993. *The Troubled Dream of Life: Living with Mortality.* New York: Simon and Schuster.

Centers for Disease Control and Prevention. 2011. "Fast Stats: Nursing Home Care." Available at http://www.cdc.gov/nchs/fastats/nursingh .htm.

Centers for Medicare and Medicaid Services. 2010. "Nursing Home Compendium." Available at http://www.cms.gov.

Crampton, Alexandra. 2009. "Global Aging: Emerging Challenges." Pardee Papers No. 6. Boston University.

Egan, Kerry. 2012. "What People Talk About before They Die." CNN. Available at http://www.cnn.com.

Ekerdt, David J., ed. 2002. *Encyclopedia of Aging.* New York: Macmillan.

Farmer, Bonnie Cashin. 1996. *A Nursing Home and Its Organizational Climate: An Ethnography.* Westport, CT: Auburn House.

Fillion, Lise, Martine Fortier, and Richard L. Goupil. 2005. "Educational Needs of Palliative Care Nurses in Quebec." *Journal of Palliative Care* 21 (1): 12–18.

Fishman, Ted C. 2010. *Shock of Gray: The Aging of the World's Population and How It Pits Young against Old, Child against Parent, Worker against Boss, Company against Rival, and Nation against Nation.* New York: Simon and Schuster.

Foundation for the Aid of the Elderly. 2012. Available at www.4fate.org.

Gamino, Louis A., and R. Hal Ritter, Jr. 2009. *Ethical Practice in Grief Counseling.* New York: Springer Publishing.

Gawande, Atul. 2010. "Letting Go: What Should Medicine Do When It Can't Save Your Life?" *New Yorker,* August 2, pp. 36–49.

Geertz, Clifford. 2000. *Available Light: Anthropological Reflections on Philosophical Topics.* Princeton, NJ: Princeton University Press.

Glenn, Evelyn Nakano. 2010. *Forced to Care: Coercion and Caregiving in America.* Cambridge, MA: Harvard University Press.

Goffman, Erving. 1961. *Asylums: Essays on the Social Situations of Mental Patients and Other Inmates.* Oxford, UK: Anchor.

Hochschild, Arlie. 1983. *The Managed Heart: Commercialization of Human Feeling.* Berkeley: University of California Press.

Howe, Neil, and William Strauss. 1991. *Generations: The History of America's Future, 1584–2069.* New York: William Morrow Publisher.

Irurita, V. F., and A. M. Williams. 2001. "Balancing and Compromising: Nurses and Patients Preserving Integrity of Self and Each Other." *International Journal of Nursing Studies* 38:579–589.

Jacoby, Susan. 2012. "Taking Responsibility for Death." *New York Times,* March 30.

Kaiser Family Foundation. 2005. "Health Poll." Menlo Park, CA: Kaiser Family Foundation.

Kaufman, S. R. 2005. *. . . And a Time to Die: How American Hospitals Shape the End of Life.* New York: Simon and Schuster.

Kiernan, Stephen P. 2006. *Last Rights: Rescuing the End of Life from the Medical System.* New York: St. Martin's Griffin.

Korczyk, Sophie. 2004. "Long-Term Workers in Five Countries: Issues and Options." Washington, DC: AARP.

Kübler-Ross, Elisabeth. 1969. *On Death and Dying.* New York: Macmillan.

Logue, Barbara J. 1991. "Taking Charge: Death Control as an Emergent Women's Issue." *Women and Health* 17 (4): 97–121.

Lorde, Audre. 1984. *Sister Outsider: Essays and Speeches.* Freedom, CA: Crossing Press.

Margolies, Luisa. 2004. *My Mother's Hip: Lessons from the World of Eldercare.* Philadelphia: Temple University Press.

Merriam Webster Dictionary Online. 2010. Available at http:www.mer riamwebster.com/dictionary.

Minkler, Meredith, and Thomas R. Cole. 1999. "Political and Moral Economy: Not Such Strange Bedfellows." In *Critical Perspectives on Aging: The Political and Moral Economy of Growing Old,* edited by Meredith Minkler and Carroll L. Estes, 37–49. Amityville, NY: Baywood Publishing.

National Institute on Aging. 2011. "90+ in the United States: 2006–2008." U.S. Department of Health and Human Services. Available at http://www.nia.nih.gov/.

Neysmith, Sheila, and Jane Aronson. 1996. "Home Care Workers Discuss Their Work: The Skills Required to 'Use Your Common Sense.'" *Journal of Aging Studies* 10 (1): 1–14.

Nuland, Sherwin B. 1993. *How We Die: Reflections on Life's Final Chapter.* New York: Vintage Books.

Olson, Laura Katz. 2003. *The Not-So-Golden Years: Caregiving, the Frail Elderly, and the Long-Term Care Establishment.* Lanham, MD: Rowman and Littlefield Publishers.

PBS *Frontline.* 2010. "Facing Death: Facts and Figures." Available at http://www.pbs.org/wgbh/pages/frontline/facing-death/facts-and-figures/.

Pipher, Mary. 1999. *Another Country: Navigating the Emotional Terrain of Our Elders.* New York: Riverhead Books.

Saunders, Cicely. 1990. *Hospice and Palliative Care: An Interdisciplinary Approach.* London: Edward Arnold.

Shield, Renee Rose. 1988. *Uneasy Endings: Daily Life in an American Nursing Home.* Ithaca, NY: Cornell University Press.

Shim, Janet K., Ann J. Russ, and Sharon R. Kaufman. 2006. "Risk, Life Extension and the Pursuit of Medical Possibility." *Sociology of Health and Illness* 28 (4): 479–502.

Smith, P. 1988. "The Nursing Process: Raising the Profile of Emotional Care in Nursing Training." *Journal of Advanced Nursing* 16:74–81.

SSCA (Special Senate Committee on Aging). 2009. "Canada's Aging Population: Seizing the Opportunity." Available at http://www.parl

.gc.ca/40/2/parlbus/commbus/senate/com-e/agei-e/subsite-e/Aging_
Report_Home-e.htm.

Steinhauser, K. E., E. C. Clipp, and M. McNeilly. 2000. "In Search of
a Good Death: Observations of Patients, Families and Providers."
Annals of Internal Medicine 132:825–832.

Twigg, Julia. 2000. *Bathing, the Body and Community Care.* London:
Routledge.

United Nations. 2000. *World Population Ageing 1950–2050.* Department
of Economic and Social Affairs Population Division. New York:
United Nations.

———. 2008. *Program on Aging.* Available at http://www.un.org/esa/
socdev/ageing/popageing.html.

U.S. Bureau of the Census. 2009. Census Brief: Nursing Homes. Available
at http://www.census.gov/compendia/statab/2012/tables/1250194.pdf.

———. 2010. 2010 Census Results. Available at http://www.2010.census
.gov/.

Vladeck, Bruce C. 1980. *Unloving Care: The Nursing Home Tragedy.* New
York: Basic Books.

Walter, Tony. 1994. *The Revival of Death.* London: Routledge.

Waxman, Henry. 2001. "Nursing Home Quality Protection Act."
Available at http://www.oversight-archive.Waxman.house.gov/.

Index

Karla A. Erickson is an Associate Professor in the Department of Sociology at Grinnell College. She is the author of *The Hungry Cowboy: Service and Community in a Neighborhood Restaurant* and coeditor (with Hokulani Aikau and Jennifer Pierce) of *Feminist Waves, Feminist Generations: Life Stories from the Academy.*